T0382855

BOUNCE BACK

12
WARRIOR PRINCIPLES
TO RECLAIM AND RECALIBRATE YOUR LIFE

TRAVIS MILLS

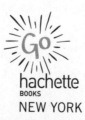

hachette
BOOKS
NEW YORK

Hachette Go, an imprint of Hachette Books
Hachette Book Group
1290 Avenue of the Americas
New York, NY 10104

HachetteGo.com
Facebook.com/HachetteGo
Instagram.com/HachetteGo
First Edition: November 2023

Hachette Books is a division of Hachette Book Group, Inc.
The Hachette Go and Hachette Books name and logos are trademarks of Hachette Book Group, Inc.

The Hachette Speakers Bureau provides a wide range of authors for speaking events. To find out more, go to hachettespeakersbureau.com or email HachetteSpeakers@hbgusa.com.

Hachette Go books may be purchased in bulk for business, educational, or promotional use. For information, please contact your local bookseller or Hachette Book Group Special Markets Department at: special.markets@hbgusa.com.

The publisher is not responsible for websites (or their content) that are not owned by the publisher.

Print book interior design by Sheryl Kober.
Library of Congress Control Number: 2023943873
ISBNs: 978-0-306-83176-8 (hardcover); 978-0-306-83178-2 (ebook)
Printed in the United States of America
LSC-C
Printing 1, 2023

*To my family and to those who have served
and sacrificed their life for this country.*

CONTENTS

Contents

FOREWORD

We all face challenges. We all have setbacks. We all suffer.

When these difficulties hit, some people break. They surrender. They let circumstances, fate, and events that unfold control their attitude, dictate their emotional state, and determine their destiny.

They adopt a defeatist attitude of negativity. They accept failure.

They curl up in a ball and wait for the clock to run out.

They quit.

But there are other people who are diametrically opposed to that attitude—people who, in spite of incredible challenges, adapt and overcome.

Of every person I have ever met in my life, Travis Mills has faced the most traumatic, intense, and brutal challenges a human being could face—and he faces these severe challenges continuously, every day, over and over again.

And yet, he has the best attitude of anyone I know or have

ever known. His emotional state is always positive. His humor is always on point. His mentality is pure strength of will.

Despite suffering the most horrific wounds imaginable, he chooses his own destiny and is unstoppable in his drive and commitment to live life.

Travis Mills is one of my friends, one of my heroes, and the most inspiring human being I have ever met.

Travis received injuries beyond all comprehension. While serving in the US Army in Afghanistan, an improvised explosive device big enough to destroy a vehicle ripped off his arms and legs, leaving him a quadruple amputee. In that moment of shock and despair, when most people would be focused on themselves, Travis's first response was to direct the medics tending to him to care for his fellow soldiers instead. He thought he was going to die. Against the odds—and thanks to the skill and determination of those medics—he lived.

But his battle was far from over. In fact, it was just the beginning. Upon returning to America, he started on an almost unbearable journey of recovery and recalibration. Countless surgeries. Excruciating pain. Hallucinations. Fighting to stay alive.

Then, he had to learn how to live again. He had to learn to utilize prosthetic limbs. He had to learn how to walk, eat, and accomplish seemingly ordinary tasks like getting dressed and brushing his teeth. He also had to recreate his identity now that he could no longer serve in his beloved Army. And, most important, he had to recalculate and reimagine how he could be the husband and father he knew his family deserved.

This was not an easy path. I cannot think of anything in life more difficult to overcome.

Yet, Travis has achieved exactly that. He has excelled in every aspect of life. He is an author, a business owner, the founder of a powerful charity organization, a speaker, and a devoted family man. He is a recognized source of laughter and light to all who encounter him.

Without question, Travis Mills has turned tragedy into triumph, and victimhood into victory. In the game of life, Travis Mills is the undisputed champion.

Thankfully, Travis is also generous—he wants to share the experiences he has had, the lessons he learned, and the protocols he utilized to overcome pain and strife and to live a life that is filled with meaningful achievement.

Bounce Back is an instruction manual—an owner's guide for the challenges of life. With moving stories of struggle coupled with his signature humor, Travis tells us how to face setbacks, how to find a path through traumatic events, and how to conquer the trials we face.

He gives us pragmatic advice on what to think—and how to think—about the misfortunes that ensnarl us. He explains how to communicate about our struggles so they do not control us. He explains the critical difference between blaming ourselves and taking accountability. He teaches us how to control our emotions and our attitude, provides a protocol to overcome fears, and educates us about the habits and benefits of being grateful.

Travis's skill as a leader also shines through in this book. He knows we need specific instructions. That's why each section has actionable tactics we can use to move forward. He tells us exactly what to do when we find ourselves playing the blame game. He gives us step-by-step instructions to follow to keep moving toward our goals. He communicates distinct options we have when we need support. He even coaches us in methodologies to help practice being more positive. This book is a road map to emulate Travis's journey past trauma and torment, onward to peace and gratification.

The book also includes experiences beyond Travis's. He shares the stories of other people who have met with catastrophe and persevered. He explores what they learned and how their knowledge can be captured and passed on to others. We read about Liz, whose husband, a B-1 pilot, was killed by a drunk driver. Suddenly a young widow, Liz had to raise two children on her own. We are introduced to Ray, a veteran struggling with survivor's guilt and a loss of identity. And we are introduced to Anna, trying to muddle through a difficult divorce. How did these people face these challenges? That is the question that Travis answers in this book.

Bounce Back is also a reminder that our human experience is not unique. We all struggle. We all feel alone. Yet, most of us think that no one could understand or relate to the discord and darkness in our lives. That is wrong. Suffering is universal. Struggle is inescapable. If anyone in the world understands struggle and suffering, it is Travis Mills.

But, luckily for us, Travis also knows there is a path through that darkness. He knows what to do and how to do it—and he shares that with us.

This book is a masterclass in recovery, renewal, and recalibration. Travis does not make excuses. Travis does not complain. Travis is not held back by challenges he faces—he is propelled forward by them. Let's be more like Travis.

Travis Mills is the best example of the human spirit I have ever known.

Thank you, Travis, for sharing your lessons with us.

Thank you for showing us how to live.

Thank you for being my hero.

Jocko Willink
May 2023

INTRODUCTION

We all have a moment in our lives we'll never forget—a moment that completely changes our life's trajectory.

For me, it was not the blistering hot day in Afghanistan on April 10, 2012, when I dropped my backpack and inadvertently set off an IED intended for a truck. It was not that day that nearly killed me and left me seriously injured, although I will say that day was a really, really bad day at the office.

No, my moment came some eighteen months later, alone in my in-laws' bedroom on a small Texas ranch. As I sat on the edge of the bed, I looked at a young soldier staring back at me from a small sterling silver picture frame. Sporting a bright orange baseball hat and a toothpaste ad–worthy smile, the soldier stood proudly in uniform, flanked by his squad, grinning in the Afghan sun.

That soldier was me, US Army staff sergeant Travis Mills of the 82nd Airborne Division. The picture had been taken only two years earlier, but it might as well have been another lifetime. I was no longer that man in the image and would never be again. That was the moment I felt helpless. Enraged. Despondent. Afraid. All at once.

And we all have those moments.

I had a hard realization: My military days were over, and I would never wear a uniform again. I would never give orders to my men again. I would not fight for my country again. I was no longer Staff Sergeant Travis Mills serving on his third tour of duty in Afghanistan. In the army, everything had been laid out for me. There was always a clear mission and a thorough strategy to execute it. I always knew what I need to do and how to get it done. Now, it was just all so... unknown.

I know I am not supposed to admit this—especially as a former member of the 82nd Airborne—but my eyes welled up. I blubbered between deep gulps of air, trying to catch my breath.

Luckily, my wife, Kelsey, walked in at that moment. I used what was left of my right arm to wipe my eyes as she sat down next to me. As soon as she saw my blotchy face, she looked into my eyes and, rubbing my back, reassured me, "Everything is going to be okay. We have each other, and you know we can get through *anything*. It's all going to be fine." She didn't say much else—she didn't have to. Just being there helped.

I knew she was right. Kelsey and my daughter had been with me every step of the way while I recovered at Walter Reed Army Medical Center. My parents, her parents, and my extended family were also so supportive. My fellow soldiers had my back (and still do). I knew I was one of the lucky ones. There were plenty of fellow soldiers who didn't get to go home. There were others who made it but didn't have the kind of support that I had. Some still carried the weight of war, which seemed nearly impossible to get past. In that moment, in Kelsey's arms, I made the conscious decision not to let the enemy win. I had to grieve for that person in that picture, or I couldn't move forward. I thought, *Okay, I am no longer that Travis. That's the old Travis. That whiteboard has been erased. I have a pen in my hand, and I can totally start anew.* I began to see life as two choices: you move forward or backward. What I wanted in my life was in front of me, not the one in that photo.

Though the man in that photo was gone, to me the choice was clear. Damn if I don't hate that I will never feel the skin of my wife's hand in mine or throw my son in the air to catch him. But there was only one direction to go, and that was forward.

Whether you are reeling from an illness, divorce, an act of violence or abuse, the loss of a job or a loved one—the list goes on—nearly everyone experiences grief and trauma in their lifetime. In fact, 70 percent of adults in the US (nearly 223 million people) have experienced some sort of trauma at least once in their life.[1] An average of 30 percent of Americans are depressed or anxious[2]—and this statistic was at the start of COVID—so many of us have experienced our own challenges in one form or another. While none of us can change what happened to us, we all have the choice of how to deal with that trauma. I am here to tell you that we are not defined by bad days; we are defined by how we *react* to those bad days. I had one bad moment—yes, terribly bad—but I won't let that one moment define me. And that moment in Texas provided that revelation. It made me realize that although I had triumphed over enormous physical challenges, I still had some big emotional ones before me. It was a decisive moment, as it made me pivot—not to the past—but to the future and all the good that was in front of me. I learned to *separate the trauma from the struggle*. In this book, I'll lay out the steps that helped me stay the course through the tough days. I'll emphasize that what matters is not *that* you struggle, but *how* you struggle.

What do I mean? Well, I would never have had the opportunity to do what I have done with my life if that IED hadn't exploded on April 10, 2012. I am not a doctor (although I have three honorary doctorates, Kelsey tells me that doesn't make me an actual doctor), and I won't pretend to have all the answers, and everyone goes through shit differently. Some will say that my recovery from the injuries I sustained was extraordinary. I wouldn't, and I don't. Just as trauma takes different forms, trauma also affects us all differently. I have picked up some great knowledge that I want to pass on. I can't take away your struggle, and I can't (literally) walk in your shoes. But I *can* show you how to struggle better. I can offer a light in the dark, a crack in a door, in hopes that it helps lead you to recovery, healing, and a life of gratitude. I will show you how, while you may have been wounded, you don't have to *stay* wounded. I'll help you instead to recalibrate.

In this book, I'll offer up the twelve principles that helped me and continue to help me through tough times. Some of these principles build on an amazing concept called post-traumatic growth, an increasingly popular and promising antidote for those with post-traumatic stress disorder. (The National Institutes of Health defines PTSD as a disorder "that develops in some people who have experienced a shocking, scary, or dangerous event.") The post-traumatic growth theory posits that a person can experience profound growth as a result of the struggles that they have experienced. I first found out about it through the Warrior PATHH, a post-traumatic growth program developed by the Boulder Crest Foundation to help those with combat experience, in particular, post-9/11 veterans, as well as first responders. I was so taken by its program that my foundation—the Travis Mills Foundation (TMF)—started offering the program as well. While the Warrior PATHH is geared to combat vets, I saw how its core philosophy could be beneficial for anyone going through a difficult time, not just soldiers or first responders. These practices can help anyone, whether they're dealing with the repercussions of an act of violence or abuse, economic hardships, divorce, or a serious illness. The strength of these concepts will be buttressed throughout the book by personal stories of people from all walks of life who have ultimately triumphed over great struggles. I know when I was going through my roughest of times, hearing about other people's handling of adversity always made me feel less alone, and these survivors have graciously opened up to me so that their success stories can be an inspiration to spur you, my friend, to read on and hopefully make positive changes in your own life.

My background is in the 82nd Airborne, but I promise this won't feel like boot camp. I won't take it easy on you, either—there is a lot of work ahead, but be certain that my practices will help you in the healing process and increase your capacity to persevere, so you can lead a productive, even happy life. I hope you find the voices in this book a chorus of hope through your own darkness.

BOUNCE
BACK

That Dog Don't Hunt

Stop Torturing Yourself and Stop Asking "Why"

In the late summer of 2020, I visited my buddy David Vobora to get a personal training session at his Adaptive Training Foundation (ATF) in Dallas, Texas. I had met David, a former NFL linebacker for the Seattle Seahawks, at a birthday party in Dallas in early 2014 when, over some whiskey, he charmed me into becoming a guinea pig for him and created a unique workout to align with my injuries. We developed a friendship, and more important, he enjoyed helping me so much that he eventually started a foundation that adapted workouts to the challenges posed by injured vets and athletes.

One of the last nights I was there, I crashed a barbecue for the twenty or so men who were attending a weeklong workshop. As the sun went down, the guys started to gather around a bonfire, enjoying burgers and beers. Someone suggested that they assess the week. One thing led to another, and the conversation got a bit heavy. Now, anyone who knows me knows I shy away from that sort of touchy-feely stuff. Not that I don't believe in it—talking about feelings in front of a bunch of strangers is just not my cup of tea. So, I made my way to the back of the group, expecting to sit out on the kumbaya moment, when one guy named Bruce, who had been injured in a car accident and paralyzed from the waist down, spoke up.

"I just have to keep going. Because if I slow down, I'll just end up crying. The worst part of it all is that I don't understand *why*. Why it happened, why it happened to me...."

Joe, the head counselor, replied, "Let's dig into that...."

Oh no, we won't, I thought.

"No. No, you don't," I said, this time aloud, my outburst surprising the group. I surprised myself too. I meant to be lying back, just enjoying the bonfire.

The counselor shot me a look and asked, "What are you talking about?"

"There is no digging into why because you're never gonna get the answer you want."

"What do you mean?"

"I get it—Bruce wants to understand why this was meant

for him. At first, I did too. But the truth is 'that dog don't hunt.' What I mean by that is, you're never going to get that answer. So, why harp on it? You are only slowing yourself down from accepting something you can't change and moving on. As I live and breathe, I will never know the answer to why I stood in the exact spot where there was an IED buried into the ground, waiting for me. It's a fight you are not going to win. Ever. So, why not make peace with it?"

There was a long silence, except for some loud cicadas beckoning from the woods behind us. I worried I spoke too much, too harshly. Some people aren't ready for the hard truth. But after a minute or so, I saw many heads nodding in quiet agreement.

Believe me, it took me a while to get to that understanding. When I first got hurt, I had a nasty case of the "whys" while lying in that hospital bed, not knowing what my future looked like. My wife can tell you, I tried to give her many opportunities to walk away—why would she want to hang around someone who couldn't wrap his arms around her? Hold his baby daughter? If you believe in the man upstairs, why was he playing such a bad joke on me? I felt like Lieutenant Dan, who lamented to Forrest Gump in the famous movie: "I should have died out there with my men. But now, I'm nothing but a goddamn cripple, a legless freak! Look. Look at me. Do you know what it's like not being able to use your legs? . . . This wasn't supposed to happen. Not to me." But nobody had that answer—not the doctors, not my family, not my buddies. None of us will get the answer to why bad things happen to us, until we enter those pearly white gates.

After a few months of the inner demons hashing it out in my head, I came to a new understanding of the old southern saying "that dog don't hunt," meaning an idea or thought that doesn't work, much like a dog that isn't very good at hunting. All the what-ifs and "Why did this happen?" only delay the ability to accept things that have happened. I decided that I had to be okay with not getting an answer. I was alive, after all—a lot of my buddies on the front lines didn't have that luxury.

This nagging feeling can drag on for many who have loss in their lives. Take Mitch, a buddy of mine whom I met through T.A.P.S., the Tragedy Assistance Program for Survivors, an organization that supports the families of fallen soldiers who died serving our country. He lost his father at a very young age, a twin sister at the age of twenty-nine, and then six months later, his nine-year-old child was diagnosed with terminal cancer. It took him a while to circle around the abyss, but he came out the other side about a year after his son's death, and now he often speaks to people around the country about grief. He uses another metaphor that works just as well: He compares asking "why?" to trying to get mercury off a table. Not only is it dangerous, but it is also so slippery that you can't possibly contain it. It is a great image that speaks to the futility of trying.

DON'T RELIVE THE PAIN

I always start my speaking engagements with a joke. It is just my nature to go for humor to break the ice. After all, there is always a bit of unease when I first come out onstage, walking on two metal legs and waving an artificial arm. There is usually a pause in the room, a collective break in the breath that always seems to take a minute to return. (I always put them at ease with a line like, "I hope this one goes well, I really bombed at my last event...." Corny right? But it works in lifting the mood.)

My body is something that people always struggle with at first meeting me, because it's a physical manifestation that says I went through something. I had something bad happen to me.

But that is it. Something bad happen*ed* to me.

Past tense.

Behind me.

I moved on.

It is that simple. One night in 2014, after my documentary premiered in Colorado, a vet came up to me, and I could tell from his eyes that he was still hurting inside. He asked me, "Tell me something... do you keep asking why this happened to you? You must think about it all the time."

I responded, "No, I really don't. I've accepted what happened and had to move on. It was hard, but I am very happy with my life and my family—life goes on."

"You're lying to me. There is no way."

"Really, no, I am not lying. I had to make a choice to move on or stay stuck. If I kept thinking of that day, I'd be reliving the trauma over and over again. I'd be retraumatizing myself. There is no way you will be able to move on if you keep reliving such trauma. I had to think of my wife and my kids, and I made that choice to move forward. It took discipline not to go there, but I knew I had to do it for myself and my family. I chose not to stay wounded."

He told me I was a liar a second time, then a third. He insisted that I was putting up a facade. I didn't like being called a liar, but I felt bad for him—his pain felt so raw. Knowing he was a vet—he may have been struggling with PTSD—I couldn't get him to believe me. Unfortunately, I have crossed paths with other people who concluded the same thing. How could I be so well adapted? I may be a bit too sunny and high-energy, but I am also proud of what I went through to get where I am today. So, it hurt to be called a liar. I hope that, in time, he found a good way to heal and come to terms with his past.

BE OKAY WITH UNCERTAINTY

Your struggle may not stem from a physical injury or illness—it could be a relationship that has ended, a death of a beloved parent, or getting let go from a job you loved. Whatever the hardship is, part of it is a loss of control over your life. It is a loss of a routine, of a life you knew and loved. You may get sad, anxious, and even angry, and it is only human to ask why, as it is in our nature to seek understanding, certainty, and closure. The human brain is not designed to handle a lot of psychological uncertainty. It can cause a lot of anxiety because, to the brain, uncertainty means danger.[1] So, it is only natural to want to have an answer. Without knowing why something happened, it may feel like a vast wasteland of unknowns stretches before you.

STOP ALL THE RUMINATION

Harping on the whys and looking for certainty is where you get into a cycle of overthinking. Without stopping that loop of questions cold in its tracks, you will remain stuck, and you will stay mad or sad—why would you want to live like that?

It will take resolve and a bit of will at first, but you need to push beyond the why. And once you do that, you can start to realize the opportunity you have before you—acceptance. That doesn't have to mean you are over it, but it does mean you can move on from it. I am not sure who said, "Use the past, don't let the past use you," but wow, truer words have never been spoken.

It isn't easy, especially for those with PTSD, which is known to bring on excessive rumination.[2] But it is necessary. I can't make yesterday not happen, just as I can't make ten years ago not happen, just like you can't make a divorce or a job loss not happen. That is part of life—but you know what? We can't always change the situation, but we can change our attitude. It sounds easier than it is, I know. But I look at it this way: No amount of ruminating will magically grow my arms and legs back (although that would be pretty cool, wouldn't it?). So, I like to say, "Don't deliberate, recalibrate." Take, for instance, the term "wounded soldier." I don't call myself that. I instead call myself a recalibrated soldier because the word "wounded" feels powerless. Like a victim of a crime or other trauma, you're a victim one time, but you don't have to be a victim for life. I was wounded once (badly), but I am not wounded for the rest of my life. So, don't become a victim of uncertainty. You cannot give it power like that, or it will power over you.

I also don't like to hand power over to fate, either. Some people have told me, "Maybe this was God's plan for you the whole time." They mean well, and if I were a more religious man, maybe I would believe it. Instead, I think, *Well, did those plans include my being blown up? Really?* Instead, I like to think that what doesn't kill me has made me stronger. This is a concept of post-traumatic growth we'll get into later in the book, but it is a powerful belief that everything we live through makes us who we are today. I am different from the day before my accident. I am stronger for it.

When people go to that place of darkness, they don't see. They can't see the future. They can't see that things are going to get better. Don't get me wrong. It is completely natural to wonder why something happened to you. It is natural to want to have an answer—good or bad, we search for the logical. We need closure; we think it will allow us to move on. We try to think through a problem to better understand it, but sometimes that brain of ours goes into overdrive and becomes an endless loop of doom. And if we have experienced some sort of major trauma, your endless loop of doom may turn into catastrophic thinking. We may feel like that event is proof that anything and everything bad can happen to us, and we develop catastrophizing as a coping mechanism, and feel in a constant state of alert.[3]

Rumination is like getting your tire stuck in the mud—you are pressing on the gas, but you aren't moving. You get frustrated and mad, but that mud is back splashing all over the truck. To get out of it, you need to think differently. For me, I figured, well, my limbs are not growing back, so I can mope about it or change my thinking. It was an active choice—and one that I continue to work on to this day—but it was a no-brainer. The alternative would not only keep me stuck, but could also become debilitating in time, causing anxiety, depression, and sleep and eating issues.[4] It can also threaten your relationships. In time, no matter how supportive your loved ones have been, they may grow tired of the negative thoughts, and they may start to distance themselves from you.

Are You Ruminating Too Much?

Some signs that you may be overthinking what happened:

Do you ponder, Why did this happen to me/my family?

Do you think, What if I hadn't done x, y, or z? Would there have been a different outcome?

Do you often wonder what life would look like if this hadn't happened?

Do you play out the accident/incident in your head repeatedly?

Do you feel what happened was unfair?

Do you blame yourself for doing something or not doing something that could have avoided the trauma?

This kind of thinking can't be turned on and off like a faucet, though. We need to work at it as we retrain our mind to stop that feedback loop. Here are a few tips that help me when thoughts fill my head:

1. Mark the time you find yourself doing the ruminating. Is it in the morning? At night, when you are trying to go to sleep? Can you spend that time

doing something more positive? Can you challenge yourself and ask why you think this way? Are your thoughts rational? Realistic? How is this serving you? Because I can promise you, it is not serving you well.

2. Do you blame yourself? What if you had only done x, y, or z? What-ifs are also nonproductive. Some people like to say that they must have been a bad person or did something wrong in a previous life to have been handed such a bad card. But really, is that rational? Think long and hard about whether these thoughts are productive, and where it gets you. If you can't help yourself, limit the time you wander. Time yourself and place a limit on how much you will ruminate. Five to ten minutes, tops, a day.

3. Talk to someone. A friend, or if you feel you need more help, find a good therapist who specializes in grief and trauma.

4. Take a good walk. Besides being a good distraction, walking outside or a bout of exercise has shown to be a huge mood elevator and clears your head.

FLIP THE SCRIPT

It is easier to see a path if you see this as a choice. Stay stuck or go forward. When you do that, then you can make a commitment to challenge that part of yourself and be intentional about doing the opposite. Flip the script. You'll need to accept that there are two things in life that we can truly control—our attitude and our effort; everything else is out of our control. No matter how bad the cards you get dealt, you get to choose how to play them. You choose how you are going to respond and how your experiences are going to shape you.

This sort of thinking does not happen overnight. It takes time, and it takes constant discipline. While I don't see myself as handicapped, there are still a few moments of my day when I need help getting my legs on, but that is the only time I legitimately give it a thought. But I'm gonna be honest with you. There are still times—maybe every four or five months—when I'll lie in bed after a long day with the lights and the TV off. It is dark and way too quiet. That's when thoughts can still creep in. I lie there, looking at the ceiling, and start thinking, "Where did I go wrong in life to deserve this? How can I still keep going in life?" I let that thought sit in my head for about three minutes. I acknowledge it. But then I think of all the good I have in my life. I have a beautiful wife and two kids who love me. I may not be able to show my son, Dax, how to throw a spiral, but I can stand next to him and coach him through it. We can't ignore these feelings, because they are real, but we can sit with them, acknowledge them, and then be intentional about flipping the script and looking toward the positive.

There will always be days (or nights) when dark thoughts creep in. How you respond is up to you. You can give room and acknowledge it, but then you have to recognize you have power over it. It's like that old adage "It's not what happens to you. It's how you react to it." It's a mindset that you'll have to practice all the time. There's no getting over it—you just have to get through it.

Take Liz, who I met through Tuesday's Children, a non-profit founded after 9/11 to help families who have been affected by terrorism or mass violence. She had been married to Steve, a B-1 pilot in the Kansas Air Guard, and they lived in Wichita, Kansas, with their two young children. One day in February 2002, because the weather was bad and his plane had been grounded, Steve decided to have lunch with their daughter Colleen, who was in the second grade. He was nearly at her school when he was killed by a drunk driver. A young widow at thirty-three, Liz had to learn how to raise two kids on her own.

The grief was paralyzing. A few days after the accident, Liz was sitting with her father, a retired marine, at the dining table, picking at a pasta dish a kind neighbor had dropped off. She asked her dad, "What if I had gone to have lunch with Colleen, too? What if he wasn't off work that day?" She continued with all the possible scenarios that could have changed the course of events.

"Sweetheart, these are questions you will never find the answer to. They will only drive you nuts and everyone around you in the process. So, decide now: do you want to be there for your kids? Or do you want to constantly try to answer the question of 'what if?'" he asked her.

She got it. "I realized I had a decision to make. And my decision was that the kids weren't going to lose both their parents that day—I decided that I needed to be there for them. I could not ruin my kids' lives." After that night's realization, Liz got help for her kids—and for herself; they were all meeting with a trauma counselor by the end of the month. "My dad was right. You can't answer the unanswerable question."

Liz had to make that decision to move forward. (I use "move forward" and not "move on" here because I think grief is something that you can't just get over. You have to push through it.) "I was once asked to define my life in six words. I answered, 'She lives but for her children.' But I also live on for my husband. Steve was an incredibly good man, and I didn't want the kids to forget about him. I encouraged them to talk about him. I wanted to create some sort of memorial for him, but my priest, a retired army chaplain, wisely warned against that. He said, 'Of course, remember him, honor him, but don't have a permanent memorial in your home because that can lead you to getting stuck in the past.' He was right. Making a living space wasn't going to bring him back. I had his folded flag from the army. I had vacation photos I could reminisce from time to time, and I had two wonderful children who inherited his amazing smile. He would live on through them. They are what stopped me from getting stuck in my grief."

LAST THOUGHT: WHAT'S THE ALTERNATIVE?

If you still feel that you are having trouble, I'll leave you with this: what's the alternative? No amount of asking "why?" will change anything for the better. It will only stop you from moving forward. And you'll stay stuck, angry, or depressed. Why would you want to live in the past when you have the ability to be better, to do better, and to get better? You can get stuck in the mud, or you can go forward. It won't be easy, because you'll be pushing into the unknown. When I was lying in that bed when I first got to Walter Reed, I was like a twenty-five-year-old baby. I had to learn how to feed myself again, brush my teeth again, use the restroom again. I could have gotten stuck right there, angry at the world, not willing to do the hard work. I could have just moved back home and done nothing but dwell on what I had and who I was before the accident. But then, I would never have seen what I could become.

Unpack That Rucksack

Process What Happened So You Can Grow from It

When I tell people to stop asking why something bad happened, I don't mean to shut the door on everything. You still need to process your experience to make sense of it. There is a difference between rumination and reflection, as well as merely overthinking and understanding.

Trauma can teach us something if you let it, so rather than just ruminating on the past, you need to purposely dissect it to understand it. With that, you can move forward and grow. Until then, you're stuck. If you had told me ten years ago that I would be thankful for my injury, I would have thought you were crazy. I was still angry, confused, and in denial. Today, while I still can't say I am grateful that it happened, I can say I am grateful for what I learned from it.

I bring up our PATHH program here because its main concept of post-traumatic growth (PTG), developed by psychologists Richard Tedeschi, PhD, and Lawrence Calhoun, PhD, in the mid-1990s, theorizes that people who endure adversity can not only get past the trauma but can often see positive growth afterward. It is the scientific evidence that backs up the old adage that what doesn't kill you makes you stronger. And unpacking your rucksack, understanding what happened, is the first part of this process. Do you like to tinker with a car or fix a broken appliance? Well, you have to remove everything and lay it all out. You have to inspect all the pieces, pick them up, and view them from different angles, looking for broken parts, before you can put them back together. It's like that for understanding the trauma you went through. You need to dissect and probe before you can rebuild. There will be some uncomfortable moments and emotions as you unpack, but the following should help you sort through what you are feeling and offer some help on how to address them.

LOSING YOUR IDENTITY

One of my PATHH guides at TMF, Ray, struggled with his identity when he left the military after twenty-seven years. He had gone into the army as a seventeen-year-old, and so when he retired, he didn't know anything different. How do you suddenly acclimate to civilian life? How do you go from 100 to 0 safely? He had a hard time shedding that identity, especially one that saw years of intense combat action and carnage. "I went through a period where I had lost twenty-two men during one of my deployments to Iraq that had been extended from twelve to fifteen months. I was angry and sad for years because I did not know how to grieve the losses or make sense of the experience. I came to an impasse. I lost my identity, and was confused about how I was still alive even though I traveled on the same roads and walked the same ground where others were killed. It wasn't like I did anything special." He eventually found the PATHH program, and by working for TMF is helping others with this same feeling of loss.

I, too, had to face my loss of identity. When I was at Walter Reed, I was busy dealing with my injuries, so my focus was on getting physically better. I pushed and pushed myself in the hospital because all I wanted to do was get out of there. I just wanted to be done with the military and live my life. But when I left Walter Reed and was officially retired, I felt that I had lost my identity. I was no longer doing what I thought I was put on earth for. I was just retired staff sergeant Travis Mills. With no direction. Nothing. Nothing going on. This was my lowest point, as I gave myself a pity party. I thought, *I'll never be as cool as I was in uniform fighting for freedom. I'll never be that badass again.* I was grieving the loss of who I was and who I thought I would be for my whole life, but he was now gone. When a therapist buddy of mine told me about the rucksack analogy, at first, I didn't get it. Putting down that rucksack is what got me in trouble in the first place, right? But a time came when I had to say, *All right, I can't go back in time, I cannot undo what happened, so how do I move forward?*

And what I realized is that I was nostalgic for one of the worst times of my life. Not the explosion, obviously. I'm talking about not eating, not sleeping, not bathing…and living in mud huts. The heat. The dry sand. The snipers. There is a saying in the military, "Embrace the suck." It is the acknowledgment of something that is extremely unpleasant but necessary. You accept it so you can better the situation. It was my job to suck it up, and heck if I didn't have a blast with my buddies doing it. Today, I see embracing the suck as an apt analogy for what people go through in difficult times. It is definitely uncomfortable and at times excruciating, but necessary to progress.

Anyway, I started using that analogy in my life. Okay, I'm never gonna be that cool. And I don't have my arms and legs. Well, that sucks. My wife is going to have to help me do a lot of things. My kids will never know what it feels like to hold my hand. It was all just overwhelming, but when I dumped out that rucksack, I realized that (1) I didn't die. That means I am alive. Alive enough to live. (2) I have an adoring wife who is going to stick by me. And (3) I have two kids who don't know their dad to be any different. I have a wonderful life. I shed that old identity and bore a new one, different. Better, cooler.

Whether you are former military, or someone who lost a job or a spouse—you may feel your identity is gone too. If you spent a lot of time as someone who had taken on a "persona"—CEO, teacher, nurse—and you no longer fill that role, it can be incredibly difficult to find a new purpose. Whenever there is a major break from a role you had carried out for years, you may have a sense of not feeling "whole." The worst thing you can do is bury that loss.

IT'S OKAY TO HAVE EMOTION

As a military professional, I know that it is hard for us service people to share. We don't let others know about our feelings because we're tough as nails, right? It is ingrained in us as early as boot camp. And well, as the popular army saying goes, shit rolls downhill. We don't like to burden others with our problems. I often use humor to deflect my feelings, so believe me, it was hard for me to unpack that bag and see what was inside. Men especially are prone not to show "weakness." But as I know now, weakness doesn't mean being emotional. Being emotional actually shows strength. In these early days, I began to realize even though I fought in Afghanistan (three wild and crazy tours), I am not Mr. Tough Guy. Not all the time, anyway. I know I need to emote. There are others who experience a trauma that is so painful, they will try everything to avoid talking about it at all, or they may avoid places or people associated with the event. But to get better, you have to do the work, and that means talking.

It is not easy. My high school friend Mike, an agronomist in the farmland state of Iowa, had been going through a tough divorce when, in the early hours of March 29, 2021, his house caught on fire. Luckily, his two kids were not there that night, and Mike and Rhys, his dog, who alerted him to the smoke, got out just in time. Hours later, his house was gone. His community around him—work, family, friends—was great. In a flash, they were there to offer support, providing him with supplies, food, and clothes. GoFundMe pages were set up to help him rebuild.

Time went by, but the trauma stayed with him. He started having dreams—well, just one, really—that haunted him every night. "Every night I would have a very vivid dream, and it would play out just like how the fire happened, but this time my kids were there. I would go to their rooms, but both their doors were shut and I couldn't get either one of the doors open. I could hear both of them crying. I'd put my ear up to my daughter's door, and I could hear her crying and pounding on the door right next to my ear to get out. Then, I would wake up. It was always this exact moment in the dream. And of course, I couldn't go back to sleep after that. Who could? I was afraid to go to sleep."

These recurring dreams wore on Mike a lot, and the lack of sleep didn't help. Friends told him he needed therapy, but he would brush them off, telling them, "I'm good." He had already been dealing with an emotional divorce and a bad bout of COVID; he figured if he could get through those alone, that there was nothing that he couldn't get through. He thought toughing it out was just going to make him a better person, a stronger person. His friends, like me, would check in on him regularly, but he kept pushing us away.

"I didn't want to talk to anybody. I realize now I was dealing with some PTSD stuff, but back then I just swallowed it and said, 'You just gotta get through it.' I was just trying to get by. But then one night around ten o'clock, I felt a sudden jolt that there was something in the house with me. I felt a huge weight on my shoulders. I didn't see anything, but it was as if a dark cloud was following me. It was a very strange feeling—and scary.

"I ended up sitting up from nine o'clock till about two in the morning. I couldn't move. I just sat there and cried. And admittedly, I had some suicidal thoughts. It was all so scary and unfamiliar—I wasn't a person that had depression or suffered from anxiety. I somehow made it through the night and called my doctor the next morning, but it still took me months to see someone.

"Travis would call me every day to talk and he'd explain to me some of the PTSD stuff that he had gone through. 'Mike, I'm telling you, this is textbook PTSD. It's not anything to be ashamed of.' He told me of his own struggles. 'I can be driving on a four-lane highway and I can see a plastic bag on the side of the road. I honestly start to swerve across four lanes of traffic because I think it's a fucking IED every time. You know, you don't have to hold everything in. You don't have to do everything alone. Don't keep in pain. There are people you can talk to about it. I'm not a therapist, but you can talk to me about it. It's better than the alternative. It's better than holding it all in to a point where you're thinking darker suicidal thoughts.'"

Mike did finally see a therapist a few months later. "I learned so much about myself, and learned the right way to handle everything. There's a stigma out there for guys with mental health issues and the wrong answer is not to talk about it. I wish I had talked to somebody a lot sooner. It certainly didn't change me overnight, but it was eye-opening to me. I thought I had been a good dad through all this, but through therapy I realized my trauma affected my kids, too. I was so afraid anything was going to happen to them, to the point I was afraid to leave the house. I always made the excuse to cook at home and watch TV. It was safe there."

He was being overly protective in fear of something bad happening. He didn't know that he was self-regulating, shoving emotions down and avoiding them, which only amplified his anxiety and exemplified that the world was dangerous. Now, talking it through with someone, he had an outlet to safely unpack his trauma and process his emotions. He realized it is okay to have issues to go through—that is life. Having them wasn't a sign of weakness; and getting help was a big sign of strength. He started to heal, and while he can't get that year back when he was traumatized, he is grateful he did get help when he did to get his life back on track. And guess what? The nightmares finally stopped.

TALK IT THROUGH

There is a lot of benefit that comes with sharing your struggles with another human: the biggest being, you find out you're not alone. When something bad happens to us, we tend to feel that we are the only ones dealing with it, and if you focus on the traumatic event itself, then, yes, of course you are alone, as you were literally the only person experiencing that very event. However, if you change your perspective and focus on what comes with the experience (depression, anxiety, anger), what you will find is that everyone has experienced similar effects to some degree. When you share your feelings, you discover that you really aren't alone. That realization alone can lift a tremendous weight off your shoulders. Now, that doesn't mean sharing with everyone you meet. You need to find someone or a group of people you trust to confide in. That someone shouldn't judge and/or try to "fix" you, but be someone who will sit and listen from the heart, to empathize and understand. (This is why Alcoholics Anonymous [AA] works so well.) Someone who will tell you what you need to hear not what you want to hear. They hold you accountable and remind you that you can hold yourself accountable. In doing this, they help change your perspective. It also gives you the opportunity to formulate what exactly is going on. Where are these feelings coming from? Are they accurate? Or is it your perception of things that is causing issues? Real-world example: Being late used to be one of the biggest pet peeves of James, my program director at Travis Mills Foundation. (You'll be hearing from James throughout this book; honestly, he is better at talking about feelings than I am, since it's his job.) If someone was late meeting him, he perceived it as that person not caring about him and not valuing his time. He would then, in his words, "instantly become an asshole." This reaction was based more than likely on a false perception. That person may have gotten stuck in traffic, spilled their coffee, had a meeting that ran over...insert an infinite number of things that go wrong in everyone's lives that would give them a good reason to be late. When we struggle, we tend to immediately jump to these false perceptions because that's what our inner dialogue is telling us. If we state them aloud, and listen to the words, we can often see how silly those perceptions are. This also works by writing our thoughts down. Read them out loud and then challenge them. Are they really true or are they just perceptions that we have created? Once we discover that we are struggling with the perception, it is helpful to figure out where that perception is coming from...because it definitely came from somewhere.

Back to the lateness example—James says this stems from childhood. Since he relied on his parents for transportation, he took it as his parents' not valuing him if he was late to school or events. Once we know where a feeling comes from, accept that it is real (no matter how invalid it is), then and only then can we take steps to stop it. This is also a process: be self-aware when we have these feelings, challenge them (are they false perceptions?), and then intentionally step outside the box and look at them from different angles. Maybe there is a genuine reason people are acting the way they are. James's parents were busy working parents trying to survive; they loved and definitely valued him. So, in reality, he was holding on to a false perception (unknowingly) from his childhood and letting it dictate his actions nearly thirty years later. Sounds super silly now, but it is extremely common. You have to unpack your rucksack to figure these things out, and it helps to share it with someone else.

DON'T LISTEN TO NAYSAYERS

There are going to be plenty of people who will give you bad advice.

"Just get over it."

"Things happen for a reason."

"Move on."

"It is what it is."

I have a friend, Anna, who was going through a difficult divorce several years ago. She was muddling through, leaning on friends and letting her work occupy her mind and time. About three months into the separation, she found out a close friend had told another friend that Anna needed to "get over it and move on." Since she wasn't part of the conversation, Anna never confronted her friend over it, but really, she wouldn't have known what to say. This was a friend she thought had her back and yet had made a really insensitive comment. It hurt her; obviously, this friend didn't know the extent of the trauma she was going through. Luckily, she had been seeing a therapist who helped her understand that the comment probably had more to do with her friend than her own situation.

It's easy for others to offer up such advice when it is not them going through it. It's a very American, midwestern attitude to have. Be tough. Get on with it. Have a stiff upper lip. So, they offer advice to push the pain away at a time when we haven't grieved in our own way, and if we listen to them, we may put up a wall so we won't feel anything ever again. But being a human is all about having emotion, so be strong and understand that others just may not understand how you are feeling.

Part of the reason people do this is that they just don't know what to say. So, we can't really blame them. But it doesn't help when we are trying to heal. They may think they are helping, but they aren't. In fact, they can only exacerbate your hurt.

Case in point: When Liz's daughter died in a car accident a few years after her husband had died, she had people say to her, "Well, your husband died. So, you know how to do this. I could never recover from the loss of my child or my husband, but you'll be okay." Those are microviolations that will only affect you if you let them. All of that is to say that you should grieve or emote in your own way. Don't let others tell you how you should feel (unless you specifically ask them for help).

IT IS OKAY TO GRIEVE

It is okay to feel. To me, grief is like the phantom limb syndrome I had in the days after my injury. My body was feeling pain in limbs that were not there anymore. They hurt; man, at times they burned like a firestorm, but why? The limb may be gone, but the pain is real. Your brain's neurons are still firing away, thinking that those limbs are still there. Even though the initial trauma—a death, an accident, a divorce—is over, your feelings, much like your neurons, need time to adapt. Much like my body's grieving for its limbs, I was grieving for my past. I was grieving for what felt normal, routine. I needed time to assess, reflect, and let go. It is often said that we don't know what we have until it is gone. Ain't that the truth? The process can be painful, but in the end, you will be on the other side and happier for it. Don't let anyone else dictate how long this process is—everyone is different and we all grieve in our own way. There is no wrong way to grieve—except not allowing yourself to do so.

What's in Your Rucksack?

When working through this process, here is a good list to keep in mind as you reflect on what is causing the struggle itself. Because if you avoid it, we can't figure it out, right? As Richard Tedeschi, one of the psychologists who coined the term *post-traumatic growth*, says, "This is the part of the process in which you talk about what has happened and is happening: its effects—both small and broad, short- and long-term, personal and professional—and what you are struggling with in its wake. Articulating these things helps us to make sense of the trauma and turn debilitating thoughts into more-productive reflections."[1]

- Find a good safe and trusted environment where you can be authentic. Vulnerable. Maybe that is with a loved one, a therapist, or a therapy group. You want a place you feel you can be yourself and empty that proverbial rucksack. To look back, to understand, not to blame, not to dwell. We need to look back so we can learn the lessons from whatever it is that we experienced and be "glad still to be here, through all the smoke, dirt and dust."

- Be comfortable being uncomfortable. Meaning, don't get used to your situation, don't accept the current scenario. Don't be afraid of going to places you don't want to go (of course, doing so with a therapist or professional is best). Sometimes, trying to remain in our comfort zone can make us miserable by not allowing ourselves to grow. Recognize what you're feeling, and let those emotions take their course. Address them, learn from them, and grow from them. You've already experienced pain, so what's a little more growing pain?

- Focus on what's in your control and what's not in your control. Let's use what is in our control to grow from it. My buddy David always says, "People, places, and things—not in our control. Our breath, our ability to see things from different perspectives, and our ability to understand that no matter what, it [all this experience, good and bad] is all for us. Those are the type of people I want to be with. Likewise, if I'm with people who can't use the scars they've been dealt to grow, then I don't want to stand by them because they're going to get hit again."

SEPARATE THE TRAUMA FROM THE STRUGGLE

Trauma is relative. Getting your limbs blown off—definitely a traumatic experience. For you, the trauma could be a car accident, domestic abuse, or an impoverished childhood. The definition of "trauma" is the act of experiencing something so distressing or stressful that it changes how you view yourself, the world, or other people in it. Whatever the trauma is—it's going to be different for different people, but the struggle is the same. So, what you need to do is to separate that trauma from your struggle. That's what we focus on.

It is the struggle that matters, and we all struggle. There's not a single person on this planet who hasn't. It's not my fault that I got blown up, but I am responsible for a good—or bad— attitude about life. This is when we need to separate trauma from the struggle.

We will have bad days, we will feel depressed, we won't want to get out of bed, we will get angry, and sometimes we react badly. That's the struggle. While I wasn't accountable for what happened to me, I am accountable for what I do with what happened.

In other words, don't let the trauma define you. You may have been a victim of a crime or, like me, wounded, but it doesn't mean you take that with you for the rest of your life. You are not a victim for the rest of your days, just like I am not wounded for mine. It's just something that happened; don't change the way you view yourself or identify yourself. If you do, you will not take back your life; instead, you will continue to feel overpowered and defenseless. You need to know that while you couldn't control what happened to you, you can control how you react. It is a mindset; that is why I don't call myself a wounded warrior. That just conjures up such a negative connotation and invites pity. I don't need anyone's pity, and I don't need to pity myself.

Once you accept that the inciting incident shouldn't define you and your future, you will see a path forward. I understand people may first see me as the guy who had a bad day at the office, but I want them to leave remembering me as "Oh, yeah, he's one of the owners at that marina, and he has a great family . . ." I want to hear the accolades of my actual life rather than my injuries. It's like the term we use at TMF: we don't use the word "tools"; we say "practices" when discussing the steps of moving forward. Tools are what you use when a car breaks down.

We are not broken.

So, it's important to separate the trauma from the struggle, and you need to see yourself for yourself, not in the shadow of what happened.

FOCUS FORWARD

Early in my recovery, I noticed a big difference between me, an amputee, and somebody who hadn't been physically injured. While they don't have anything visibly impeding them, they are still hurting; their pain is just harder to detect. I could more easily focus on recovery because mine was physical, but it's harder for people who don't have something to point to and say, "This is where it hurts." But they hurt all the same, and they don't know why. So, then they feel stuck, and they find themselves looking in the rearview mirror.

We use the rearview mirror analogy often during the Warrior PATHH retreat at the foundation. It's pretty much a bunch of strangers when it starts, but within 24 hours, they share their deepest thoughts. Since it is a safe place, they feel comfortable saying whatever they want to say. But in between hard things, we have them do some lighter things to give everyone a break, like archery or meditation. On the last day, they look back one last time. It's where we introduce them to the analogy of the rearview mirror, borrowed by the two founders of the PATHH program, Ken Falke and Josh Goldberg. The concept is rooted in the idea that you are in the driver's seat and want to move forward. The rearview mirror—representing the trauma in your past—is only there as a reminder. You can check it every once in a while, but you don't want to stare at it. There will be days when you need to look, to remind yourself of where you have been and how far you have come; you may even slow down, and revel in that distance, but avoid looking at it all the time, or you will not be able to progress and finally see past the struggle.

There will be more bumps in the road, but make the choice to keep driving forward.

What do those bumps look like? For me, I still wish that I could do things with my kids. Everyone once in a while, I will see another dad wrestling with their son, and I'll have a

Stop Comparing

We have a bad habit of comparing ourselves to others. We do it in nearly every aspect of life, and we also do it when it comes to our struggles. When James started as an intern at TMF, he judged himself for being on the struggle bus. He looked at vets who had much more physical impairment, and thought to himself, *Here is someone whose situation is so much worse than mine and yet he's doing great. What do I have to be "messed up" about?* He held on to that mentality for a long time, and it did two things:

1. It caused him to judge himself even more harshly than had before.

2. He put whomever he compared himself to on a pedestal, which put a sense of pressure on them to be "perfect." That person has now been given expectations to live up to, and if they make a mistake or have a bad day, then they feel they are failing the people who look to them for strength. This perpetuates the idea that they can't talk about their struggles, which is counterproductive to growth.

moment when I think, *Wow, that sucks. I can't do that with Dax [my son].* That is looking in the rearview mirror. There is certainly an acknowledgment of, "Ugh, if I only had one arm or one of these limbs, how much different my life would look..."

But then it's gone. Because I can't do anything about it. It doesn't stay with me. I stop looking in the rearview mirror. I had my moment of vulnerability, and I let it go. I worry more about those who never show that vulnerability because they've ignored it. At some point, it's going to rear its ugly head.

I love this quote from Bessel van der Kolk, MD, in one of the best books on the subject of trauma, *The Body Keeps the Score*: "Nobody can 'treat' a war, or abuse, rape, molestation, or any other horrendous event;...what has happened cannot be undone. But what can be dealt with are the imprints of the trauma on body, mind, and the crushing sensations in your chest that you may label as anxiety or depression, the fear of losing control, the self-loathing...the nightmares and flash-backs....Trauma robs you of the feeling that you are in charge of yourself..."[2]

To me, unpacking your rucksack is the first step in getting your life back. A close second is having compassion for yourself.

Point the Finger, and Three Fingers Point Back at You

Don't Blame Others, and Be Compassionate to Yourself

My program director, James, knows how low one can go before getting better. A heavy equipment operator in the Marine Corps from 2009 to 2013, part of his job was dealing with IEDs during his two deployments to the Helmand Province of Afghanistan. Over time, he got used to the explosions, but still, some were worse than others. One particular blast knocked him unconscious; he was okay, outside of puking all night afterward. *Nothing to see here*, he thought, but when he got back from that deployment, his wife thought otherwise. Like any good marine, he ignored the idea of there being something wrong, whether from the IED blasts, the loss of friends, or any other number of things that he experienced. He deployed again to avoid hard conversations with his wife about his mental health. It wasn't until he came back from his second deployment in 2012 that he knew something bigger was going on.

"I was super angry. I woke up pissed at the world. And that's just the way I stayed 24/7, I didn't know why; I just knew that I was pissed. I was getting violent at work with junior marines, and verbal fits at home just kept escalating. This, among other things, ultimately led to divorce. I left the Marine Corps in April 2013—but at that point, I had been diagnosed with PTSD, TBI [traumatic brain injury], and a bunch of other crap, and was forced to seek treatment. Doctors put me on a zombie cocktail of medication—eventually, it came to a total of seventeen different meds. Some for depression, some for anxiety, some for TBI-related headaches, and a bunch of other pills to counter the side effects of the medications." His dad suggested that he move back in with him and his mother, and he took him up on it. He didn't trust himself to sit at home with his thoughts, so he started working in his dad's grocery store. He started at the deli counter, but after throwing a 20-pound ham at a customer, he got moved to the bakery. It was around this time that he felt the meds were not for him, so he stopped taking them.

Instead, he started drinking—heavily—which fueled his

anger. He swung between going out, drinking too much, and starting fights to the other extreme of staying home. On the days he stayed in, he could barely get out of bed. While he had the wherewithal to realize that going out drinking was probably not a great idea, it didn't stop him from being violent with family members and friends, blaming his actions on his TBI and PTSD. It was a vicious cycle—he knew it wasn't good for him, but he didn't know how to stop "being an asshole"—his words, not mine. He started feeling out of control. No matter how mad he was at himself, he'd instead project that anger on someone else. He'd think, *Who am I gonna blame today? Because it can't be me.* That's a victim mentality.

All this anger and self-defeating behavior was eating at him and he started to go down a darker path. "I wasn't put on this earth to hurt people, never mind the people who love me the most." Suicidal thoughts consumed him, which is pretty common in the military—veterans are 1.5 times more likely to die by suicide than nonveteran adults.[1] Like many of them, he felt it would be easier on his loved ones if he just wasn't here, walking on this green earth. One night, in a split-second decision to take his own life, he drove his truck off the road, and made it 100 yards into a thicket of woods before hitting a large rock. He walked home, took a nap, and then called the cops. "I felt like I couldn't do anything right—I can't even kill myself right."

What did finally go right was that the accident was the wake-up call that James needed. He knew he needed to figure things out. He joined a veteran's motorcycle club—it became a place to talk to people with similar experiences. It was a slow process, but it was a step in the right direction. He soon came to terms with the anger that he placed on others. "I realized I didn't even know what fucking emotions were other than anger. We can't be so caught up with our wounds that we become oblivious to other person's feelings or emotions." The biggest aha moment was when James realized he was accountable for himself. "If I don't change my [metaphorical] diaper, then I'm going to have shitty pants. That's on me. I stopped looking outward to blame and started to look inward." As he went through his own rucksack—meaning he processed what happened—he slowly came to terms with the fact that he was a changed man, and that he *could* choose *how* it changed him. He found an appreciation for life and for the people who tried to help him.

Eventually, James went back to school for recreational therapy and ended up doing an internship at my foundation, and now he helps folks like himself on their journey. (Apparently, he only learned about TMF because his grandmother was a big fan of mine—she even had pictures of me on her refrigerator, more of me than James. . . . I am not kidding.)

WHY DO HUMANS LIKE BLAMING OTHERS, ANYWAY?

Well, the scientific explanation is called "projective identification." We unconsciously put unwanted feelings (projection) onto people around us (identification).[2] In other words, when something goes awry, we tend to put the blame on others. It's a defense mechanism. And typically, we lash out at our favorite people. James was displacing his anger, and he placed it onto the ones he cared about the most.

This blaming will only lead to anger, resentment, and broken relationships if you don't take a hard look at yourself. Here is what you can do when you find yourself playing the blame game:

1. Acknowledge when you are doing it. Are you unfairly projecting blame onto a family member? Spouse?
2. Sit with it. Ask yourself why you are feeling the way you are, and is there any way to look at the situation differently? Know that you are in pain, angry, sad, or whatever emotion is bringing you down, and be compassionate toward it. It's legitimate. Don't bury it and don't stiff-upper-lip it. Just like you wouldn't ignore a friend in pain, don't ignore it in yourself.
3. What can you do today to lessen the pain or the anger? Can you call a friend to talk it through? Walk it off?

DON'T BLAME YOURSELF

Now, let's turn over that blame coin. Just as you shouldn't pass the blame onto others, you should not blame yourself. I know a lot of vets who rake themselves over the coals for something they did or did not do in combat. Maybe they didn't reach a wounded friend in time to save them, or weren't fast enough to accomplish a mission. We soldiers are trained to perform at a high level. From boot camp on, we had it beaten into us with the no-BS attitude of "pick it up, you piece of shit." Now, this was done so that when the real battle shit hit the fan, we listened to our commanding officers, no questions asked. Nonetheless, this browbeating could lead some to feeling "broken." The military is not the only place where you can have that feeling ingrained in your psyche—maybe it was a parent or partner who made you feel "less than." We don't even need a real person to make us take a nosedive in self-esteem. We have social media to thank for that, with Instagram posts and TikTok videos that have distorted our realities of what life should look like. With any situation of self-doubt, you need to be self-compassionate. Meaning? Have your own back.

It is human nature to blame ourselves. This tendency goes haywire, however, when someone experiences trauma—it puts everything into question, and in efforts to maintain those scales of justice, one usually blames themselves rather than upset their perception of the world. When Anna's husband, Jake, told her that, after six years together and one year of marriage, he wasn't "into it anymore," she was devastated. They were still receiving wedding gifts in the mail, after all. How could it be that he wanted to end it so soon, without trying? She blamed herself for his reversal of feelings. Of course, something had to be wrong with her, not him, she thought. It was only after several months of therapy that she could see that she wasn't to blame. Her therapist was able to show her that, as a recovering alcoholic, Jake was still processing and probably repressing deep-rooted issues that were projected onto her. In time, Anna could see the situation objectively and was finally able to move forward with her life.

Liz, whose husband was killed by a drunk driver, is a perfect example of how to avoid the blame game. "You can kind of go down a dysfunctional rabbit hole, especially when people ask me, 'Why did nothing ever happen to the man who killed your husband? Doesn't that make you angry?' And my answer is, it makes me nothing. Because he does not get any real estate in my brain. He took enough for me. He doesn't get to take one more second of my peace. I am entitled to still be happy and successful in whatever way that looks like. Could I blame myself? Sure, I could go down that road—why didn't I go with him that day? What if this, what if that... it doesn't change what happened, and I can't self-flagellate myself for something that was beyond my control." Liz was able to separate herself from the trauma of losing her husband and choose not to play victim, which would only have prolonged her trauma—instead, she allowed herself the space to grieve while being there for her children. She continued to be in control of herself—it was a deliberate choice she made. She understood that blaming herself or the drunk driver would not bring her husband back.

So, don't blame others, don't blame yourself, but hold yourself accountable. There is a difference between accountability and blame. While James wasn't to blame for the TBI and PTSD, he is accountable for his actions afterward. I, too, needed to be accountable after my accident—what if I had sat in bed with a poopy diaper on and had a bad attitude about life? Liz was accountable for her actions after the death of her husband; she had to be strong for her kids. If she blamed the man driving the car, she would have been too busy doing that instead of being there for her children. Or, if she blamed herself, she would have been doing what the therapists call personalization—when you think you are responsible for your situation, but you're not.[3] It is a need to rationalize your bad feelings—because you *must* have done something to deserve this, right?! Wrong.

Shame vs. Guilt

For the most part, when we blame ourselves, it's because we are feeling guilty about something that happened. But there can be a feeling of shame mixed in as well. Brené Brown described the difference between the two the best: Guilt is "I did something bad," and shame is "I am bad." There is a sense of unworthiness that is attached to shame that you somehow caused it to happen. You may feel shame because of how you view yourself—as weak, useless, or bad. Shame is harder to treat because, at its core, it is about self-esteem. People who experienced abuse and childhood trauma can feel a lot of shame, as their self-esteem, or lack thereof, was shaped by the abuser.

Then there is survivor's guilt, which can be an issue with people who have PTSD, which is a big issue in the military, or who experienced or witnessed a traumatic event and survived when others did not. A buddy of mine from Maine, Bob, joined the Marine Corps right after high school and did eight years of service, mostly as a helicopter crew chief (someone who maintained the craft and made sure it was all-systems-go come liftoff). He left the military in 2016, but coming home was a hard transition. "I didn't really know what my purpose was. I did eight years in the Marine Corps and had many near-death experiences. I found some work in aviation, but I was still finding it tough to find my feet. From everything that happened in the military, one of the biggest things that was tough to swallow was when one of my best friends was killed in a helicopter crash. So, I had some has really bad survivor's guilt, but I wasn't addressing it. I just looked back on the all near misses that I had, and kept wondering, *Why? Why wasn't I killed?* I didn't talk to anyone about it, even my wife. I bottled things up for a long time—I never really wanted to admit I had an issue going on." It took a few years, but Bob eventually got to the Warrior PATHH at the Boulder Crest Foundation. Unfortunately, it was a little too late to mend things with his wife, but he was happy to meet other people who were struggling with a lot of the same guilt he had.

I know this self-blame—the "should coulda woulda"s that play in our head when they want to mess with us. I had a case of it, too, as I sat in Walter Reed for eighteen months. But ultimately, I realized that while life took an unfortunate turn, my actions would decide the fate of my ultimate destination.

DON'T BE A VICTIM

You may have already come across this quote by psychologist and Holocaust survivor Edith Eger, from her book *The Choice: Embrace the Possible*, but if you haven't, here it is: "Suffering is universal. But victimhood is optional. There is a difference between victimization and victimhood. We are all likely to be victimized in some way in the course of our lives....It comes from outside. It's the neighborhood bully, the boss who rages, the spouse who hits, the lover who cheats, the discriminatory law, the accident that lands you in the hospital. In contrast, victimhood comes from the inside. No one can make you a victim but you.... We become victims not because of what happens to us but when we choose to hold on to our victimization."[4]

It is easy to be caught in the web of victimhood—we are, in a way, wired to. Our brain tends to lean toward victimization. Yeah, it's true: When we start to blame others, we start acting like a victim. You know the outdated saying "Good things happen to good people"? Well, this is a bias that has seeped into our collective psyche, so when something bad happens to us, we think, *Well, I must have done something to deserve it.* This theory, called a "just-world bias" is where victims of trauma—say rape, crime, or abuse—are blamed for their own misfortune. And while it comes from our human need for things to have a reason—that the world is fundamentally fair—that is just plainly untrue. But built-in bias is not easy to undo, and until we can right the wrongs of the world, the only person who can stop it from becoming a never-ending cycle is you.

Unfortunately, many former vets get stuck in this victim mentality. James is a perfect example. "I was an asshole when I got out of the Marine Corps for a long time, and I blamed everything I did on PTSD. I couldn't understand how some other guys died, and I was still walking on this earth. Fuck, why didn't I die? Why did the guys behind me get hurt, and I didn't? It took a lot for me to get to the place where I am today, but what started it for me was reading [Austrian psychiatrist and concentration camp survivor] Viktor Frankl's *Man's Search for Meaning*.[5] There is a quote in the book that reads: 'Everything can be taken from a man but one thing: the last of the human freedoms—to choose one's attitude in any given set of circumstances, to choose one's own way.'

"Literally, everything was taken from him, including his name. But he still called choice 'a freedom.' He chose who he was going to be throughout that entire ordeal. That human freedom exists regardless of what you are experiencing. You don't have to let your situation dictate who you are."

In other words, we can CHOOSE to live in the past and ruminate, and if we can choose to do that, then we can choose not to as well. Again, this isn't easy, but trust me in knowing that this is the right path to take if you want to move forward.

If you stay stuck in that victim mentality, you'll never be free. You may even develop what is called "learned helplessness"—a psychological term for people who feel that they have no control over their life. They don't take any actions to make their life better, even though they are capable of making them, because they are convinced that their actions have no impact. Look at it this way: Frankl may have been held captive by the Nazis, but he still saw he had freedom of choice with his outlook. You can too. It may take a bit of time to come around to this mentality, and before we can do any of that, we HAVE to accept two things.

First, you have to accept that you are being a victim. When James read Edith's quote, he realized, "I did all those things." Then you have to make a commitment to yourself to be different, to challenge that part of you and be intentional about doing the opposite.

I was a victim of an IED explosion; James was a victim of PTSD. But I decided not to play that game. I see it as I was victim*ized*—past tense. Something happen*ed* to me. Once. If I continue to let it happen to me, then I become a victim in life. That just plain sucks. So, don't perceive yourself as a perpetual victim. This tendency for "intrapersonal victimhood"—when someone has an ongoing belief that they are a victim—has the danger of becoming part of their identity, as indicated by one study done by the University of Tel Aviv.[6] And Scott Barry Kaufman, a prominent cognitive scientist, agrees: "Those who have a perpetual victimhood mindset tend to have an 'external locus of control'; they believe that one's life is entirely under the control of forces or the mercy of other people."[7] That just sounds like such a heavy burden to carry around, doesn't it? Don't let your trauma define you.

Second, hold yourself accountable for your actions. No matter what the circumstances, you are defined by the way you respond to challenges. David Vobora likes to say this isn't "the trauma Olympics." When things get difficult outside of you, it's easy to point and blame. And this is the reason that the three fingers pointing back at you are really the ones in your control to work on.

BE ACCOUNTABLE

Robert, a buddy of mine I know from the vet network, had a great city job in Chicago, and he and his wife were eagerly waiting for the birth of their first child. In 2020, he had just put a down payment on a bigger home to accommodate his growing family when his boss asked him to lunch. As he was eating his burger, his boss turned to him and said bluntly over his arugula salad: "I have to let you go." He couldn't believe it. He had no idea that this was coming. He knew things had been tough, and his quota was down, but he felt blindsided. But he kept his cool and said, "Look, you know, I accept responsibility for everything that you're saying, I want a chance to be able to prove myself, and I'd like to do that. You're the boss, and I'm the employee. This is on me that this wasn't managed appropriately. And I'm sorry for that. Can you give me some time to fix it? I'm happy to work for you at no cost, give me three months…"

Guess what? They gave him that chance. The fact that he thought on his feet so quickly showed great resilience, although he did say that was the easiest part of this story. The actual day-in, day-out grind of proving himself was harder than that conversation, but he swallowed his ego, kept his eyes on the prize, and got to keep the job after the three-month probation. He responded to a challenge with accountability and commitment to see something through; he changed his circumstances through his actions.

BE SELF-COMPASSIONATE

Compassion—sounds warm and fuzzy, doesn't it? Actually, giving yourself some self-compassion isn't that easy—because it means you need to sit with the pain, not suppress it.

When Mark Barden's son, Daniel, was murdered at Sandy Hook Elementary School in Newtown, Connecticut, in 2012, little did he know this tragedy would spur a long-term friendship with then Vice President Joe Biden. Biden, for his part, had known what profound grief felt like, having lost his first wife and daughter in a car accident in 1972 and then, in 2015, his son Beau to cancer. Over the years, Biden would often call and check in with Barden, knowing what he was going through. One piece of advice stayed with Barden: Biden told him to get a notepad and leave it on his nightstand. At the end of every day, he suggested that he mark how the days rated, from 1 to 10. "In the beginning," he told him, "most days will all be 1's, and then you'll start to get better days. The low days will always be low, but eventually, the low days will start to spread out."[8] It is a great exercise to keep yourself in check, give yourself a moment of self-compassion, and also be grateful for progress.

There are going to be days when you don't move forward (perhaps we are stuck on number 3 or 4, as in Biden's notepad). Sometimes that is the goal. Success is not simply doing better today than you did yesterday—sometimes that could mean just holding your ground. Early on, when you're just starting to figure shit out, it takes a lot of self-compassion to say, "Hey, you know what? I didn't get up and go to the gym today. But I got out of bed." Maybe you made it to the couch, right? Maybe you washed your face, right? It's a big step for someone who is in the tunnel of the struggle.

How to get yourself some self-compassion? Kristen Neff, a renowned psychologist who coined the term, recommends reminding yourself of these three elements of self-compassion[9] when you need it the most.

1. Self-kindness vs. self-judgment. You want to give yourself the same kindness you would a friend or loved one when you are suffering, rather than berating yourself with self-criticism. "Self-compassionate people recognize that being imperfect, failing, and experiencing life difficulties is inevitable, so they tend to be gentle with themselves when confronted with painful experiences rather than getting angry when life falls short of set ideals."[10] So, in other words: give yourself a break. Don't be so hard on yourself.

2. Common humanity vs. isolation. Remember that all humans suffer—that feeling of connectedness to a universal human trait should make you feel more connected, not isolated. When we feel isolated and cut off from others, our well-being takes a hit because of this evolutionary need to feel safe. "Therefore, self-compassion involves recognizing that suffering and personal inadequacy is part of the shared human experience—something that we all go through rather than being something that happens to 'me' alone."[11] Bottom line: to suffer is to be human.

3. Mindfulness vs. overidentification. First and foremost, you have to be aware of your suffering to be able to be compassionate. Rather than avoidance, you need to recognize and acknowledge your pain so you can give yourself the care you need. The constant self-criticism of not being good enough will only drown out the hurt. You'll need to pay attention to what is going on, observe and describe your experiences, but do it without judgment. Also, be careful of the balance, here—you don't want to identify with it *so much* that it consumes you and you become completely immersed in your pain, losing all perspective.

If you can give yourself this kind of compassion, it will go a long way to helping you build resilience.

While you're at it, **give others some, too.** This isn't just about compassion for ourselves; we need to have compassion for others. It is a great skill to have to be able to put yourself in other people's shoes, a skill that is becoming a lost art. But when you have compassion for others, real communication and connection happen, which will only make you—and your relationships—stronger. It will also give you a sense that no one struggles alone.

FORGIVE

This is a big one, especially for those who have been traumatized by a violent crime or abuse. How do you forgive someone who has done such a horrible thing to you? For me, do I forgive whoever put that IED in the dusty soil in Afghanistan in 2012? Well, they were doing their job and we were doing ours; it was a war, after all. But no: I can't forgive. I can't be like the WWII hero Louis Zamperini, whose life was chronicled in the best-selling book *Unbroken* by Laura Hillenbrand.[12] Though he forgave his tormentor, nicknamed "The Bird," and other captors in his two and half years in Japanese POW camps, I can't turn the other cheek. But for others, it may be possible. This is one time where I step aside and not clamor on, because I think this is such a personal decision. But here is a question to ask yourself to help you figure it out: Would forgiving the person who did you wrong help you move forward? Some say that forgiving puts too much emphasis on the abuser, not the survivor,[13] so you'll have to work it out on how it feels to you.

I have a friend, Laura, who was a victim of sexual abuse when she was in college. For years, she held it in, and she didn't even tell anyone about the incident, for fear of being shamed or blamed. Years later, she still couldn't shake her own shame, though, and she finally saw a therapist about it. A few months into it, she was able to write a forgiveness letter. It wasn't sent to the perpetrator, but the act of writing out all the feelings and thoughts was enough to let Laura feel that she could finally move on from the experience.

"It was long after the incident, so writing the letter wasn't so much out of anger; I wrote it more to get rid of this nagging feeling that what had happened was keeping me from moving on. I wanted to stop thinking about it. So, I wrote the letter to him, explaining what I had experienced and how he made me feel, but I was done it having control over me. And most importantly, I forgave him. It was so cathartic, because, while the event itself was traumatic, I realized there were things about it that made me stronger because of it. The mere fact of writing all this emotion down let me put it behind me. At last, I didn't feel shame or feel like a bad person. It was so freeing."

So, reader, you may be asking yourself right about now: If the letter was never sent, what happened to it? Did she keep it?

"I took a match and burned it. Over the toilet. Living in a city apartment, I don't have a fireplace, so there isn't much choice where I can burn something. But it seemed oddly appropriate to do so. Then I flushed it. Bye, bye."

Swoosh.

There may be times when you may need to forgive yourself. If you have trouble forgiving yourself—after all, we discussed earlier about blame and accountability—remember a great line in Mitch Album's classic memoir *Tuesdays with Morrie*, about his old professor dying of ALS: "It's not just other people we need to forgive. . . . We also need to forgive ourselves."[14]

Essentially, everyone has regrets for things they did or didn't do, but you can't get hung up on these regrets, or you will never get peace.

None of this is going to happen overnight. But this practice of self-compassion will help if and when you start to rake yourself over the coals when something bad happens. This self-flagellation is counterproductive to the process, so remember: you WILL fall down, but if you continuously beat the crap out of yourself every time you do, getting back up is going to be almost impossible.

So, repeat after me: "I am human and I make mistakes." Show yourself some grace, accept the mistakes, and LEARN from them. Instead of dwelling and letting them hold you back, use them to propel yourself forward in a new direction. Life is trial and error; there is no handbook on how to live your life. Every time that you feel you may be beating yourself up, stop, reflect on the situation, and ask yourself: "What can I learn from this situation? How can I do better?"

It takes time to learn that blaming others or yourself is a useless exercise; instead, giving yourself self-compassion is the way to go. It won't be a quick fix, but it is a journey you will be happy you took. At the TMF, we interview people before they come to do our PATHH program. We do this because if we feel the veteran is stuck in a victim mentality, they are not quite ready for the program. We know that if they came, we would be setting them up for failure. There is a right time and a place—you need to work on being ready for that in your journey. When I woke up in the hospital bed, I knew I had to make a choice. And that choice was that I wasn't going to be victim. It was an easy choice for me, but for others, it is a harder road. For James, it was a messy, overly long trip. How does he feel now? "I generally have a good attitude, I am able to let things slide. I don't really care what other people think about me. As long as I'm happy and the people that I'm close with are happy, then I'm good. I see it in the people that I help [at TMF]. The biggest thing that's helped me the most is self-compassion."

Snap Your Fingers, Wiggle Your Toes, and Get the F*** Out of Bed

Create Small, Achievable Goals for Moving Forward

Anyone who knows me will tell you that I am probably the most impatient person they have ever met. Poor Kerry, my physical therapist at Walter Reed Hospital, would be first in line to tell you so. The first time I went down for rehab at MATC (Military Advanced Training Center) in May 2012, I made quite an impression.

"Hi, I am Travis," I said, barely letting Kerry speak before I continued in my 100-mile-an-hour cadence. "What's the fastest a quadruple amputee has ever been out of here? Because I'm gonna beat it."

"Whoa, welcome…," she said, "I love your motivation… but I don't care how long you're here for. I am here to just make sure you get everything out of us that you can so that once you leave, you don't ever have to come back. With the extensive work we need to do, I think we are looking at about three years."

"Well, I am going to do it in nine months. I have a wife, a daughter…I got a family to take care of, things to do…," I told her breathlessly.

Kerry patiently told me otherwise. My goals—while inspirational and lofty—needed to be a bit more realistic. In the days that followed, I realized she was totally right—this was not something I could do quickly. My body could only be pushed so much. I was at the mercy of a healing timeline: I needed to be able to stand up before I walked, and I needed to walk before I ran. I needed the patience to let things heal. Baby steps that cannot be avoided, skipped, or raced over.

Mind you, I am still not that *good* at patience—I hated the days and weekends I couldn't work on my body, but I got through it. I did so by making measurable and achievable goals.

I wanted to be able to walk again, feed myself, and eventually drive—all things I took for granted before my injury. So, Kerry and I discussed how to make goals for myself that were realistic. My first goal was to walk again, which I did in two months' time—a feat in itself because my new legs felt like they were made of cement.

My goals were challenging in their own right, but they were physically based. For those who may be dealing with an emotional injury rather than a physical one, setting goals works just as well. People dealing with PTSD may find it harder to create goals and stick to them because the condition is known to affect motivation,[1] but doing so will help them recover better. Achieving goals also provides hope and boosts confidence, as well as gives a sense of accomplishment.[2] They will motivate and challenge you to do even more goal setting. It may not be immediate, but let me tell you that you can do whatever you put your mind to. Goals can be a measuring stick for progress, and when dealing with adversity, any small step forward will feel like a huge feat, especially in the early days.

A SIMPLE CHOICE TO ACT

Admiral William H. McRaven made making your bed—a simple task—a profound act of achievement in his best-selling book on leadership, *Make Your Bed*.[3] Now, you may be in a state where, before you can make your bed, you must make the choice to get out of it. When dealing with trauma, there may be days—weeks—that you don't feel like doing even that. You may feel so depressed and deflated that you are too paralyzed to do anything. That, my friend, is called collateral damage.

To which I say, snap your fingers and wiggle your toes. I can't do that, for obvious reasons, but chances are that you can. The idea behind it is simple—do one small thing to get you moving. That one small thing will get you motivated to go on to the next thing—the simple act of getting out of bed. And getting out of bed will curtail whatever you got spinning in that mind of yours. The mere physicality of these actions should spur a mental shift as well. Once you stop being physically and mentally stuck, you can start to take responsibility for your behavior. Choose to see something in your life that you can find a positive in every single day. Snap your fingers, wiggle your toes, get out of bed—it's a simple act that can remind you that life isn't that bad. These may sound trivial at first, but they can be very intentional, deliberate ways to start doing something that is positive. Getting out of bed is a specific, measurable, actionable, and realistic act. No matter how small the act is, the choice you are making to move forward is huge.

BE S.M.A.R.T. ABOUT IT

When I was sitting in Walter Reed feeling like a failure for being a casualty of war, I blamed myself for having that IED go off, letting everyone down. But I also like a good challenge. I wasn't about to let my condition as a quadruple amputee ruin my life. I felt that it was daring me to succeed. It was as if my body was saying, "Come, I dare you to work with this."

And so I did. And I instinctively—well, with a little help from my therapist—took incremental steps to prove to my body I could do it.

Goals and Feelings of Failure

This feeling of failure I had is extremely common for most people who struggle. No matter how out of our control the situation may have been, we generally tend to feel like it's our fault when things don't go the way we had wanted or planned. This is extremely important to recognize, especially when setting goals, because if we don't meet one, we feel deflated, which tends to send us backward, instead of forward. Sometimes people will just quit altogether. This is why we have to be intentional about setting realistic goals.

Taking a series of small steps—believe me, my body wouldn't allow me to do more—led me to eventually sit up, stand up, walk a lap, then three laps, then a mile. All these microachievements eventually lead to a big improvement. So, I believe goal-setting is a huge factor in anyone's recovery—physical or emotional. To come up with these marginal (and maybe not so marginal) goals that will help you accomplish what you want to do—maybe it is finding a new job after being fired, or sticking to a sobriety plan—it takes S.M.A.R.T. goals. S.M.A.R.T. was created in the 1980s as a business leadership strategy to plan and execute goals, but it has since been co-opted by the military, and it works for "real" life, too. I have science to back me up: Studies show that people who have specific goals are more likely to stick to them than those who don't have specific ones. In an analysis done on goal-setting research, 90 percent of the studies showed that "challenging goals led to higher performance than easier goals, 'do your best' goals, or no goals."[4]

So, what does S.M.A.R.T. stand for?

S is for Specific: What is it that you want to accomplish or get over? Narrow down your goal as much as possible. For me, it was to walk three laps in two months.

M is for Measurable: Give it a quantifying marker. Want to run a marathon? Is there a specific race you would want to qualify for? What is the time you want to do it? It will help you keep on track if you have something that is measurable to know whether you have achieved it or not.

A is for Attainable: Your goal has to be feasible and achievable yet pushes you out of your comfort zone. My goal of getting out of Walter Reed in nine months was not feasible in the time period I initially set for myself, but working with Kerry, we figured out that eighteen months was much more doable.

R is for Realistic or Relevant: This is to make sure your goal has purpose and that it has value. This is about finding your why—why do you want to do this? For your kids? To get ahead? For your health? Having a motivating reason will help you stick with it during challenging moments.

T is for Timetable: You'll need to give your goal some sort of time frame or time limit. If you have a goal without a timeline, you will inevitably slip—you won't have the accountability to finish and you'll likely procrastinate. Be it a week, a month, or a year, a time frame will help you keep on target. If you were too ambitious and missed your deadline, just reassess and readjust.

Remember, take one step at a time. Make one actionable goal and build on it. It's about setting attainable goals now that you have made the decision to move forward. Some days, that may mean just having one good productive hour. The next day, it may be two. Success is not necessarily doing better today than you did yesterday. It can mean holding your ground and not doing worse. When you're just starting to figure shit out, that takes a lot of self-compassion to realize that just staying in one place is good enough, and that can give you enough optimism to look forward to the next day.

Keep on Track

Once you have a goal, you'll need some tips to keep you going.

1. **Be flexible.** Did you miss a day? Did you accomplish less than you were supposed to? Don't get all bent out of

shape—just start over the next day. It is a marathon, not a sprint. Katy Milkman, a Wharton professor and author of *How to Change*,[5] explains that adaptability is actually better than rigidity: "If we want to form the stickiest possible habits, we also need to learn how to roll with the punches, so we can be flexible when life throws us a curveball. Too much rigidity is the enemy of a good habit."[6]

2. **Be kind to yourself.** In the "Principle #2" chapter, we talked about being self-compassionate. Keep doing it. This trait will help you as you set up and try to achieve your goals. Kristen Neff, the preeminent researcher on self-compassion, sees it this way: "We know from research that the number one reason people aren't self-compassionate is that they are afraid it will undermine their motivation."[7] But Neff believes that kind of thinking is wrong, and she points to the number of studies that showed when college athletes were taught self-compassion, their athletic performance improved.[8] Perhaps it is because, without some self-compassion, you may feel defeated more easily if goals are not met. And that may lead you to lose motivation. When we misstep, it is important to give ourselves some grace, understand that life is not a straight line from where we are to where we want to be. It has twists and loops, ups and downs, and is a journey to be enjoyed, not dreaded. Don't give up on a goal, no matter how small, because you didn't achieve it the first time. So, give yourself a pat on the back for even trying.

3. **Don't judge.** We are our own worst critics. No one can judge or beat us down like we can. Take a minute and think about a close friend or family member whom you care about. Think about how you would treat them if they came to you with a problem or they were struggling. How would you respond to them? What would you say? More important, HOW would you say it? What's your tone like? Once you've done that, flip the script. How do you treat yourself when you are struggling? What do you tell yourself? What's your tone like? Was there a difference in how you treat others versus how you treat yourself? If so, why? What factors or fears come into play? Now, reflect on what your life might be like if you could treat yourself the way you would a close friend. If we treated others as we treat ourselves, we wouldn't have anyone in our lives, because 9 out of 10 times we are super tough on ourselves. And while being tough can be a source of motivation, there is another way: we can motivate ourselves just as effectively without beating ourselves into the dirt.

4. **Be patient.** Yes, I need to remind myself of this, too. Daily. There is no magic button. You can't diet for two days and lose 10 pounds. Things take time. When it came down to my trying out my prosthetic hand for the first time, it took days and weeks and months to get proficient, but every day was definitely in the right direction. And the reason I knew I had to get better

was that my family was still depending on me, and I didn't want them to be feeding me for the rest of my life.

5. **Visualize achieving your goal.** I believe that visualizing something you want to happen will help it come to fruition. Now, I am not talking about wishing you were a billionaire. I am talking about realistic goals here, okay? There have been some promising studies on visualization in athletics and the business world,[9] but I am a big believer that visualizing any goal will help you get there. Maybe it is crossing the finish line, getting that new job, or for me, standing up so I can finally look straight into my wife's eyes once again.

6. **Have a support system.** We'll get into the importance of a buddy system a bit later, but know that having someone who is either a role model for you or with whom you can be accountable is huge in goal-setting. As *The Power of Habit* author Charles Duhigg asserts,[10] having a support network is so motivating when we are trying to improve. There are two main reasons for this: first, we typically get positive reinforcement from people close to us, which is motivating; and second, when we watch someone around us achieve something, it can be as if a little motivator switch goes on in our own head and we think, *Well, if he can do it, so can I.*

I first saw how pivotal this could be while I was still early on in my recovery. Marine corporal Todd Nicely, another quadruple amputee, came in to meet me one day in my hospital room. As he sauntered in with his prosthetic legs and arms, he greeted me with, "Hey, man, welcome to the club."

"I won't be in your club." Salty, I know.

"It's a kind of late now, don't you think?" he replied. Good comeback.

"You got me there," I conceded.

I asked him if he wanted a ginger ale, but he misunderstood me and thought I had asked him to get me one. He walked over to the six-pack that was stashed under my bed, squatted with ease using his prosthetic legs, reached for one, opened it was his prosthetic fingers, put a straw in it, and placed it on my tray.

"Here you go," he said nonchalantly.

"How did you just do that?" I asked incredulously.

"You will make it through this. You'll be fine. Life isn't over. It's altered, but it's not over."

From that moment onward, I thought, *Okay, if this guy can do all this, so can I.*

7. **Celebrate the wins.** Release that feel-good chemical dopamine in celebrating a job well done. Didn't stay on track? Maybe it is time for a shift in perspective or change up your goal.

8. **Reevaluate and reassess.** If you haven't successfully achieved a goal you made for yourself, go back and read through the letters in the S.M.A.R.T. acronym. Was your goal specific enough? Doable enough? Did

you give yourself a realistic timeline? Sometimes all you need is a slight shift in thinking to get something done.

DISCOVERY LEARNING

The day after I had walked three laps at MATC—about two months after the blast—I was very sure of myself. The next day, my dad came for a session as the day's cheerleader.

"I'm gonna walk five laps," I told him. "I'm gonna show you how quickly I can recover."

But as I got halfway around the track, my legs cramped up, and I couldn't move. I got super frustrated with myself, but the constant pushing of my body had hit its limit. I felt my eyes well up. "I am so sorry!" I apologized to my dad. "I can't walk any farther. I just can't do it." Buckling halfway through the walk, I felt that I had let my dad down.

But the next day, I went farther. And the next, and the next. It was a series of mini-wins that got me to walk finally. And I learned it was this series of progressions that I had to go through to get to where I needed to be.

In physical therapy, it's called discovery learning. The therapist lets the patient figure it out (whatever "it" may be) rather than somebody just always giving them the answers. All failure is a learning opportunity—in all different facets of our lives.

Making goals and achieving them will always involve making some mistakes along the way. Mistakes are good. You learn from them. It may feel like something takes forever, but if you attack each small goal with enthusiasm and passion, you will see how quickly those small achievements add up to big change.

BITE-SIZE CHANGES

Be careful in taking on more than you can chew, as the cliché goes (but it is true). Make a lofty goal into a series of smaller, bite-size, achievable changes. If you are not doing them, they're probably not small enough. For example, you want to run a marathon. Break it down to a 5K and then a 10K first, giving yourself the space to lead up to the larger 26-miler while still giving yourself the room to step out of your comfort zone. And if you succeed at doing the 5K, you'll be encouraged to go on to the 10K, which will give you the confidence to keep going and, boom, finally hit your marathon goal.

In 2012, I had made my own running goal: there came a day when I was able to dress myself again (for the most part), drive again, and eat again. But it took time and hundreds of smaller goals that led up to those bigger achievements. When I got to that space of being more self-sufficient, I made another goal. I wanted to do something *big*. I wanted to run a 5K—well, walk a 5K. I had become friendly with a bunch of 9/11 firefighters, and they were planning to do the Tunnel to Towers

5K, which commemorated Stephen Siller, a firefighter who lost his life that horrific day in New York City in September 2001.

"Hey, we're all gonna run the 5K in September," one told me. "We can push you..."

"Nope, I can do it." I hadn't had my legs that long, but no way was I going to have guys push me. I wanted to do this. They looked at me incredulously.

"Well, yeah, but we can help you—it's no big deal."

"Nope, I'm just gonna walk it." End of discussion.

That September, I traveled up to New York City, and with Kelsey at my side, I met my pals at the starting line. I was first buoyed by adrenaline at the start of the race as I limped through the first mile, but on the second, I could feel my right leg starting to feel raw.... I started to bleed inside my socket. I thought, *I've met a goal. I've walked over two miles now. I can stop... boy, I am tired. UGGGGHHHH... My back hurts....* But I kept going. I came hopping out of the Brooklyn Battery Tunnel, and as the sun beamed down, I squinted and eyed hundreds of firefighters in their gear among a vast throng of spectators with banners commemorating lost men, cheering us all on. I thought, *Well, if these guys and gals can go down this flight of stairs, risking their own lives to save others, I can finish this.* And I did. I was hurting. My body was beaten up, but I finished it. And achieving that goal was worth every sore minute.

Stay Within the Guardrails

Manage Your Emotions and Control Your Attitude

One day, I was helping my wife empty the dishwasher. I was running late picking up my daughter, Chloe, from soccer practice, so I started picking up the silverware in bunches. (Aren't I a good husband for unloading the dishwasher?) Mind you, since my recovery and prosthetics, I can pretty much do anything anyone else can, but just at a slower pace. Something that may take you three minutes may take me ten. Or fifteen. I shouldn't rush. But this time I was rushing, and my robotic hand let me down, and suddenly a cascade of silverware crashed to the hard linoleum floor. First, I was glad they weren't knives.

Then, I turned. "You gotta be kidding me," I huffed. I know it was my own fault. Can't I just grab one at a time? It is a simple task made harder with still learning how to use my hand, and it is those simple tasks that sometimes get the best of me. Life events big and small come at us every day, and it's hard not to get angry or discouraged. For me, everything was frustrating at the beginning of my recovery: I needed help using the bathroom, I needed help getting fed, brushing my teeth. But anger never solves anything: shouting or screaming doesn't get a job done quicker or faster.

People frequently ask me if I still get angry, and of course I do. But I like to say that I have bad moments, not bad days. Believe me, a quiet rage can grow inside me some days. It's okay to still get angry. It's okay to show emotion. I may have a lot of metal in me, but that doesn't make me a robot; I'm still human, right? No matter how resilient we become, life won't stop being *life*. But it's how we deal with those emotions that is important. After all, emotion is energy, and energy are emotions. So, when we are attuned to where we're putting our attention, we can manage our emotions and feelings. When we lead by our emotions and our feelings—meaning we haven't taken governance over them—we get into trouble. In other words, you want to lead your emotions; you don't want emotions to lead you.

And there are a lot of emotions—sad, happy, anxious, mad...America's Sweetheart therapist Brené Brown has identified eighty-seven emotions in her best-selling *Atlas of the*

Heart.[1] But I am a simple guy, and I want to limit this chapter to anger, because I think this is the emotion we most struggle with when we talk about resilience. (She does compile those eighty-seven into three main buckets: happy, sad, and pissed off, so I'm addressing the third group.) Many people can carry a steady, low-boil anger—whether it is anger over the situation they are in, anger over who may have caused them harm, anger at themselves for not dealing with it, or anger for how their lives have changed. That is a heck of a lot of anger to carry around. And sometimes that low simmer can get aggravated by a slight tripwire, and all of a sudden you are boiling over with rage.

I have often found myself in moments of frustration—it could be as simple as unloading the dishwasher or dropping a can of soda with my robotic arm as I try to get into my car. In those dumb but maddening moments, I can let my emotions overwhelm me OR I can choose to take back control. There are bigger moments that more than justify our feelings—a job firing, a sudden loss of a friend. Small moments or big, the takeaway is always: *You can't always control your situation, but you can control your attitude.* And if you handle things with anger, you only feed that anger. Life is still going to happen—and you will inevitably get frustrated or pissed off. But to be resilient, you will want to stay within those guardrails. In our TMF program, we define those guardrails as a mostly positive state, moving forward and keeping your cool while you travel through those peaks and valleys. You stay within your lane, keeping your emotions in check—you don't want to veer too far over to the right, with anger or a deep dive into pity, guilt, anxiety; or worse, on the left, keeping those emotions bottled up. What do I mean? Many former military personnel have trouble showing emotions *at all*—it's so drilled into them to not reveal any feelings that many of them lost the skills to access emotions, and so they can often feel adrift out in the real world. A lot of that is caused by PTSD, which can lead to emotional dysregulation, a fancy term for the inability to manage emotions due to long-term distress and trauma.[2]

Many abuse survivors have the same issues. Too much or too little emotion for too long is a dangerous road to go down. So, setting up those guardrails is a great step in helping you on your journey of resilience.

DYSREGULATION

One of my PATHH guides, Ray, whom you met in the "Principle #2" chapter, is an excellent example of someone with dysregulated emotions. He grew up with a WWII vet father and parents who both went through the Great Depression—it was a household that repressed a lot of emotion. Then, he went off to military life himself, where he "managed my emotions so much I had none." There is a difference between management and repression, and his was a learned behavior that would serve him well in the military. But in real life, not so much.

He retired from the army in 2010 as a command sergeant major with a long list of decorated combat experience, much of it in Iraq. During his tour in 2006–2007, twenty-two paratroopers were killed in action, and eighty-six were wounded. He and his commander had to visit the morgue each time a soldier was killed. They would be the last people from their unit to see the remains prior to them being sent back to the States. Ray and his commander would salute every one of them. It was a ritual that would haunt him for years. "I couldn't process my emotions," he said. "I not only knew all the men personally, but in most cases, I knew their families too. Since I was in charge of people, it was difficult to process the losses; I needed to stay focused on being a leader and our mission."

When Ray arrived home, he wasn't the same. Three years later, he retired from service, but he had a hard landing back into civilian life: the stoicism that served him well in the military didn't do him much good on the outside. "I had all these emotions because of what I saw and what I did, but I had no guidance on how to work with them." He started to realize he didn't have as much control over circumstances as he thought. He struggled with anxiety and tended to self-isolate, staying home with his wife and avoiding social situations that would make him feel uncomfortable. He wasn't dealing with a host of feelings that were boiling within him.

"I had trouble regulating my emotions. One minute, I'd be sitting at the kitchen table, eating a meal with my wife, and the next, I'd start crying or I'd get angry and stay angry for several days. It obviously served me well on the battlefield and even in difficult training, but when combined with the trauma I experienced in the military, things started to fall apart," he said. "I had to put an act on; I would go to work and act as a certain guy, but when I wasn't at work, I was struggling." Ray would go four or five days without sleeping, which resulted in chronic pain. When he drove, he would instinctually look out for IEDs; he was hypervigilant and often had nightmares. Most noticeably, he said, was the change in his relationship with his wife. "I was volatile, but I also felt numb, when I would say 'I love you' to her, I didn't have that feeling of love like I had in the past. I knew I loved her, but I didn't have the ability to feel it."

When Ray sought help from mental health providers, their protocol was to prescribe medications. Ray and his wife agreed this wasn't what was best for him, as there didn't seem to be a long-term plan to get off them once he was on them. He used medication for a short time but wanted to get to the root of the issues, so he tried different types of talk therapy off and on from 2010 to 2017. The therapy proved to be ineffective— they just weren't accustomed to treating combat veterans at the time. Ray practically begged his doctors to tell him a way to shut down his brain so he could just relax, even for just a minute or two.

In 2014, he and his wife moved from Kentucky back to Farmington, Maine, but the move didn't help—at first. There weren't any combat veterans around that he knew, and so he still felt a sense of loneliness. He moved from job to job and continued to struggle. Fast-forward two years and Ray found his way to my foundation. He started volunteering at TMF, which finally gave him a sense of belonging and camaraderie. Once TMF started offering the PATHH program, Ray jumped at the chance to attend. It helped him uncover so much of what was stopping him from living a life he wanted to. After unpacking his past, he realized he had been carrying around an enormous load of stress his entire life. He had grown up in a volatile home, and then he went into a career where he was jumping out of airplanes and experiencing combat. The high-octane lifestyle kept his adrenaline and other stress hormones riding high, which stayed that way for years. This constant heightened state of alertness caused emotions to become out of whack, or unregulated. But with the program, he learned a variety of wellness and regulation practices and began to reconnect with himself and other people. Finding a source of community and belonging, he was able to regulate his feelings in the absence of medication—to calm himself. Showing emotions—and shedding actual tears—was something that Ray learned was okay to do. For Ray, it was a community, a connection to self and others, and a renewed sense of purpose in helping people that finally helped him; but for others, it could be therapy or medication—it is the act of finding that source of support that is crucial.

Emotional dysregulation can show up differently in people; some will shut down emotionally and stay silent, pushing people away; or, on the other side of the spectrum, some get overly emotional, becoming extremely angry and volatile. If not addressed, our emotional derailment can lead to a slew of self-sabotaging and numbing behaviors, such as eating disorders, drug and alcohol use, and even verbal and physical abuse, all efforts to quell the disorienting feelings we have.[3] All these can be attempts to regain emotional control, but ultimately, they can cause more out-of-control behavior.

GIVE YOURSELF A DIFFERENT PERSPECTIVE

When Robert, whom you met in "Principle #3," was in grad school, he took an adaptive leadership class that has always stayed with him, and it came in handy when he was in danger of losing his job. At that moment over lunch, he had so many emotions consuming him. "I really want to scream, 'Hey, you set me up to fail. You didn't even communicate what you wanted from me...' I felt we didn't have an agreement on what I was supposed to do, yet here I was being told I failed. But I didn't scream. I remember what I learned in that class: to get on the balcony. Get up high and look from above at a situation. Get that perspective to get out of your head and leave your emotions on the floor, so you can be more objective and resist having a hasty reaction. Going up on the balcony gave me the space and the presence of mind to get a broader picture and figure out a good plan forward. There may be something you want to say, but that doesn't mean you should say it, and being on the balcony gave me that time to think on my feet and respond the right way."

CHANGE YOUR ATTITUDE

While more complicated or deep-rooted issues with trauma cannot be helped without therapy, one of the simplest things you can do to change right now is to change your attitude. And how you do that is a good indicator of whether you're struggling well or not. We're going to struggle regardless. That's what life is. All of the things we discuss in this book are generally impossible without an attitude change. Plain and simple. But it's not something I can teach you to do—it's something you need to do on your own. It's like if you wake up in the morning with a poopy diaper on (metaphorically speaking) and don't change it, then you're going to sit in your yucky diaper all day. Either you are going to sit there for hours, angry, or are you going to do something about getting out of that situation. You have to hold yourself accountable. You have to decide whether you want to sit in dirty diapers for the rest of your life or not. If you decide not to, you are saying to the world, *I can't change. I am just going to exist like this, forever in my angry bubble.* To be honest, that doesn't sound like much fun. What's it going to be? Want to stay and remain angry, bottled up, and mad at the world? If yes, okay, that is your choice. But I would rather not be a casualty of my own emotions.

ACCEPT THE EMOTIONS

This is a hard one for a lot of people. I get it. And I am not here to say don't be angry. I say be angry, don't push it away. Think about *why* and *when* you are angry—and *how* are you taking that anger out—and on whom? Then ask yourself, "What's it doing for me except making me *more* angry?" Accept that you have anger—after all, something put you in that position to be angry in the first place. In *The Body Keeps the Score*, Bessel van der Kolk mentions how the neuroscientist Joseph LeDoux and his colleagues "have shown that the only way we can consciously access the emotional brain is through self-awareness, i.e., by activating the...part of the brain that notices what is going on inside us and thus allows us to feel what we're feeling...the only way we can change how we feel is by becoming aware of our inner experience and learning to befriend what is happening inside ourselves."[4] For Ray, he knew no one should be in the position of having to salute and place posthumous medals on countless body bags. For me, sure, I was angry about that IED waiting for me to drop my rucksack. We each came to terms with our emotions differently, but once we both acknowledged it and became self-aware as to what we were feeling and gave it value, we could start the process of managing it. We learned to use it to our advantage: we didn't use it to fuel negativity; rather, we used it for moving forward and doing good instead. Some people will say, "There is nothing I can do about it." Scratch that: Yes, you can. Use it as a great motivator to build an internal dialogue that turns fits of anger or repression of anger into emotional management—not repression. Here are a few ways to unlock and moderate our emotions.

Breathe

Breathing is the first step in helping us calm ourselves. Your breath is linked to your parasympathetic nervous system, which controls your flight-or-fight response. During a tense moment, breathe in through your nose for the count of 4, hold for 4, and breathe out through your mouth for the count of 4. Repeat three times to slow your heart rate and refocus. You will immediately note the effect of your breathing as it calms your parasympathetic system.[5] The more you focus, the more benefit you will get from it. Notice the air in and out. You will feel calm, I swear.

Whenever I think my anger is getting to a level that I just can't accept, I do these five steps:

1. Do the breathing technique of 4-4-4.
2. Recognize your feelings. Are you angry? Are you anxious?

3. Ask this question: "Is this feeling helping me?"
4. If it's not, continue breathing 4-4-4 until the moment passes.
5. Appreciate that you got yourself out of an uncomfortable moment. It works!

Practice Mindfulness

Like breathing, mindfulness is a great way to calm yourself down from a hot mental space. Mindfulness is simply paying attention to the moment, being self-aware and nonjudgmental as you observe your emotions as they are. Try this: Breathe as spelled out in the previous technique while trying not to think about anything else but the in-and-out of your breath. If you find your mind wandering, always bring it back to the breath. You want to be aware of what is going on and be in the present moment without judging. That's mindfulness. Studies show that this simple act of reflection can help you monitor your feelings and help calm you. In fact, a recent study shows that just one meditative session can help lower levels of anger—crazy how that is, right?[6]

Meditation and mindfulness are often conflated. But how I understand it is that meditation is a more formal way of practicing mindfulness. Whereas you can do mindfulness anywhere, anytime, meditation is done in a more controlled and structured environment, often guided by a teacher. Someone once explained the difference to me: Mindfulness is being aware of your thoughts, and meditation is letting go of them. While meditation is not for me (my form of meditation is the opposite—I just keep moving! I was never one to sit still), I do know a lot of guys who live by this. This doesn't have to be done at a fancy yoga or TM studio; just sit quietly somewhere and focus on your breathing. David Vobora, whom you met in the "Principle #4" chapter, is a big proponent of mindfulness and meditation. He helps out a lot of marines at his foundation, and he often teaches many of them these practices. Here is a typical initial conversation:

"Hey, so we're gonna do some mindfulness work before we work out today," Brian says.

"Oh, so we are going full-on hippie, right?' the marine responds.

"Ever shoot between breaths when you were behind the scope of a rifle? Well, that's mindfulness."

"Ohhhh…okay, cool."

In training, marines are taught to shoot between breaths and heartbeats. That's a mindfulness practice; they just didn't know it. Heck, I didn't know it. But we were taught to breathe in 4 and out 4, which helped us naturally calm our stress in the moment, and also have our body as still as possible. The science behind this is that you are creating a dance between your sympathetic nervous system, which puts your body on high alert (a.k.a., your flight-or-fight response), and your parasympathetic nervous system, which helps you relax your body.[7] The two systems work together to keep the body in balance, so a soldier can be able to stay present and ground himself and then engage differently when he needs to—for instance, when the enemy shoots. It is a flow state that's actually calm, cool, and collected. The soldier then can show restraint by managing to hold back the trigger and fire rounds when necessary: no, no, yes, yes, no, yes, all at a very, very incredible pace. Their circumstance and soldiers' attention supersede their emotions at the pivotal moment—if they get outside the guardrails, that is where they can mess up. That's why this ability is so important—to be able to calm ourselves and ground ourselves—so that we can respond differently and better to our situations.

See the Humor in Things

Growing up, I was known as the clown in my family. I was always teasing everyone, especially my kid brother, and always getting into something I shouldn't, so much so that a recording of my dad yelling, "Don't, *Travvvvissss*!" became a ringtone on my grandfather's phone. Today is no different. I love to make people laugh, and these days, it's usually at my body's expense. Humor is even more important when things are tough. It just lightens up the room, lifts the tension, and releases much-needed endorphins in the brain, which helps de-stress. A public speaking engagement or a meet-up with kids does not go by without me rotating my wrist 360 degrees or pretending a leg falls off by accident. Initial shock is followed by chortles of laughter, and everyone has a brighter day. The joke isn't important—it is the break from whatever is running through our mind that we are going for here.

Use Anger as a Motivator

We talked before about how anger itself isn't bad—it is a valid emotion, but instead of turning it into something destructive, why not make it something that is constructive? Anger can in fact be a great motivator, a force to inspire you to do something, to change something, to make something happen. We used anger all the time in the army—maybe we were in a firefight and had been outwitted and cornered by the enemy. Everyone is angry—but we'd put that anger in the right place and at the right time, and pump ourselves up and outmaneuver the enemy. Otherwise, reactivity can cause bad decisions, and that is when soldiers die in battle.

Role-Play

In our program at TMF, we teach people how to regulate their emotions so that they can respond— rather than react—to situations, better connect with people, and better deal with daily issues. Because if you're a bull in a china shop, nobody's gonna want to be around you, right? So, a lot goes into how to we do that, and we often start the first meeting by asking them if any of them have a difficult conversation they need to have—be it with a girlfriend, wife, child, whoever. And then we role-play it. They put themselves into somebody else's shoes, and by doing so, they learn behaviors that will help them have that conversation in the real world. Often when we go through trauma, we think that nobody can know what we've been through, right? Nobody knows what combat is like except for other combat veterans, but everybody knows what struggles are like. For Ray, he didn't realize his wife also experienced trauma in that she helped wives of soldiers who didn't come back grieve. At funerals, she held babies who wouldn't know their father. She did all of this while also working as a trauma nurse in an emergency room. After learning all this, he was able to connect with his wife in a way that had long been dormant. Once you start to break that barrier and realize that you don't have a monopoly on struggle, you will see that you are not so alone. Understanding that we all go through it teaches us something—it teaches us to appreciate life and the people in our lives a bit more.

Give Yourself a 5-Minute Time-Out

When my emotions get the best of me and I feel some rage coming on, I give myself a 5-minute time-out. I go out for a walk, a drive, play ball with my dog. It gives me a break from the situation to get some fresh air and some fresh perspective.

For some, journaling and writing can better help with the processing of emotions. Some people like to take a journal with them so they can jot down thoughts and feelings as they go about their day. Some like to journal at a specific time of day; for instance, if writing at night, they might try to recapture all their feelings and thoughts from the day—how the day went, what angered them or what made them happy, why it made them so, and what they did about it. Is there anything they would change if they could? You get the gist. It helps putting all that on paper. Just five minutes can do a world of good.

Sometimes, writing in the heat of the moment can help too. I have an old friend, Meghan, who drafts an email when she is upset with someone or a situation. She types out all her thoughts in black and white but never presses Send. (Tip: She doesn't dare add an email address, just in case.) The act of writing down how she feels is enough for her. Her frustration wanes, she sees the situation clearer, and she can move past it. No matter how you use those five minutes, doing so will help you lower the temperature a bit so you can come back with a clear head.

Shift Your Thinking

I am in no way a woo-woo kind of person, but I do know that when we change our focus from the negative to the positive, it shifts our way of focus immediately. Are you mad someone hasn't paid you on time? Are you pissed off that someone cut you off on the highway today? Upset that someone undermined you at work? Take those negative thoughts and instead try to remember some good that came out of today. Had a great chat with your daughter or son? Great feedback from your boss at work? Even something as simple as having a great workout at the gym—all can help remind you that not all is bad. Turn worst-case scenarios into best-case scenarios. It is amazing how turning a thought around can lift the weight of your anger in minutes. And always go back to yourself. If you focus on yourself, everything else—those external things you can control will still happen on their own. You don't have to even try to control that. Put all of that energy into making you the best person you can be. You'll see when you have this attitude shift that things start to happen—you start to thrive.

One amazing way to help shift your thinking is to give thanks for all those good things in your life.[8] Well, hold on, buddy—that is what the next chapter is for.

Take Five

Make the Time to Be Grateful for What You Have

"**B**low (Oh-oh-oh-oh-oh-oh-oh)....This place about to blow (Oh-oh-oh-oh-oh-oh-oh)!" pumped out of the speakers that vibrated along with the song's vibrant baseline. I turned the Kesha hit up before turning around and announced in my booming voice to all in the rehab room, "TEN-SECOND DANCE PARTY!" I proceeded to raise my arm and shake my crutch in the air.

It was late 2012 and I had been at Walter Reed for about four months. It was getting a little stale, so I decided to take it on myself to add some dazzle to the morning rehab session and call for a ten-second dance party. This impromptu jig was so popular that I made it a regular thing (much to the chagrin of the staff), dubbed Kesha Friday—or Monday, or Tuesday— whenever there seemed to be a cloud of doom in the room. If one of the guys seemed frustrated or was having a bad day, I wouldn't stop until I got a grin from him. It sounds silly, but (a) I do really love Kesha, (b) who doesn't like a dance party, and (c) everyone's mood was lifted in those ten seconds. It spurred a moment of gratitude for being alive and to be able to dance—whether that was lifting our arms in a wheelchair, raising a crutch, or just bopping our head to the beat. It was a gratitude for being alive and sharing the common respect and appreciation for music.

"Gratitude" is a self-help catchphrase these days, and between you and me, I used to think it was a lot of hogwash. But now I understand how pivotal a role it has in being resilient. Case in point: There are five minutes every day I can't wait to be over: the five minutes in the morning when I get dressed, or should I say, when my father-in-law helps me get dressed. Yes, I said father-in-law. If you told me fifteen years ago that I'd be saying good morning to him every day, before saying it to my wife, I'd have thought you were crazy. Yet as surely as my buzzer goes off on my alarm clock at seven a.m., Craig is a constant, showing up every morning to help me put on my legs. He then helps me put my shirt on and buttons me up (I still can't do buttons). Once my legs are on, I stand up. He then helps with my arms. We've managed to get this routine down to a tidy five-minute routine. Although I will always dislike those five minutes—it is a constant reminder that I am indeed handicapped—I am also very grateful for them and for my father-in-law. I will gladly accept his help. Every. Day.

There is so much gratitude to go around for those people who support me—my family, my therapists, and now, my staff at the foundation. For me, gratitude came easily. I had always had a sunny disposition, which has had a mixed reaction my whole life, but I know there are many who may have hard time with being thankful or seeing the brighter side of things, especially when going through a particularly rough time. Who can see the sunny side of things when things seem so...dark? Well, knowledge is power, and there have been many studies that show us why we humans like to torture ourselves so much.

SCIENCE LESSON #1: WE TEND TO BE NEGATIVE NANCYS

It helps to know that we humans are hardwired to be negative (although I'm not sure how I missed out on the gene)—we focus more on our mistakes and bad experiences than on the good things that have happened. It's called the negativity bias; we tend to remember (and dwell on) stressful negative experiences more than the positive, and to base our behaviors off them.[1] For instance, many of us will remember a dig someone said, rather than praise. It is in our nature. Back in the days when we were hairy, knuckle-dragging cave people, our very survival was contingent on our negative reactions. Running away from a bear or tiger, spitting out a bitter berry (which was most likely toxic), or avoiding a poisonous snake—it was our body doing what it does best: surviving. This is our sympathetic system, discussed in the last chapter, at work. Nowadays, with Whole Foods and zoos, we don't need to be on constant alert for what will kill us, so we focus on smaller, more insignificant things. Traffic. Cold coffee. A coworker's dismissive email. Even with the smallest slight, we get anxious, dwell on it, and hold on to it. We can't seem to let things go. And those who have gone through trauma, particularly childhood trauma, will have a harder time since they are often playing with an overactive response system. It's not that they don't want to, but because of the trauma their nervous system is used to being in, their body is constantly on edge in that heightened flight-or-fight state.[2] So, for some, gratitude will not come easy. But with a little practice, we can stop ourselves from stepping back into dark shadows and instead lean into what is good around us.

SCIENCE LESSON #2: THIS IS YOUR BRAIN ON GRATITUDE

Studies have shown that practicing gratitude can have incredible results on the brain and mood—people have reported feeling happier, more motivated, and more content after adding the practice into their daily life.[3] It does so by shifting that heightened alert system that had been turned on ever since trauma or microtraumas—the one responsible for the flight-or-fight response (the sympathetic nervous system)—and turning on our calming (parasympathetic) system, which slows the heart rate and relaxes the body.[4] We also get a boost of joy juice because our brain releases the feel-good neurotransmitters dopamine and serotonin as well as oxytocin.[5] It's a cocktail made for happy hour.

SCIENCE LESSON #3: GRATITUDE BREEDS RESILIENCE

The more you do it, the better you will be, as well as the more resilient for future adversity. Being thankful is not going to stop shit from coming at you like some Marvel superhero, but what it will do will help you manage the rough times all the better, because the more you work on it, the more you are equipped to depend on this go-to for calming your system, seeing the positive, and keeping you moving. Studies show that consistent practice will train your brain, much as a habit will do, into being more optimistic and more compassionate,[6] which makes you more resilient. Win-win!

SCIENCE LESSON #4: REALLY BELIEVE IT

Andrew Huberman, PhD, a neuroscientist and professor at Stanford School of Medicine, made me realize something else really cool. On his *Huberman Labs* podcast, he mentioned that for it to be really beneficial, you need to believe it.[7] So, when doing these practices, I want you to believe that you are thankful for three things. Why? Well, as Huberman explains it, we have a part of the brain (the prefrontal cortex, for those who need to know) that provides reason and comprehension and perseverance: Basically, this area of the brain makes sense of everything, and it is wired to it to a deeper part of the brain that is more reactive to sensations. He continues that if you went into an ice bath because you wanted to reap its benefits, yes, it will be freaking cold; that part is something your brain can't change. But since you are doing it willingly, specifically because you know of its health benefits, the medial prefrontal cortex kicks in and prompts positive reactions to happen, such as dopamine to be released and other health effects. Contrast this to someone throwing you in an ice bath, or you are only doing the Polar Plunge on New Year's Day because your boyfriend is forcing you to: your body will have a different reaction. As Huberman explains it, your "medial prefrontal cortex is the knob, or the switch, that can take one experience and allow us to frame it such that it creates positive health effects." The opposite happens with something we don't want to do—we get negative health effects.[8]

PUTTING GRATITUDE INTO PRACTICE

Okay, Professor Mills's science 101 class is now over—you are out in the real world. What do you do? How do you integrate gratitude into your everyday life?

Be Grateful for Your Past

You can't erase what happened in the past, as they do in the movie *Eternal Sunshine of the Spotless Mind*. Nor should you want to. It's always a part of you; you just need to change the way you look at it. So I say, turn it on its head and be grateful for it. What do I mean exactly? When I was doing research for this book, I came upon Anderson Cooper's podcast that he did about grief. (I know, I listen to a lot of podcasts.) Cooper, grieving over losing his mother, Gloria Vanderbilt, and having lost his father when he was a teen and his brother to suicide when he was in his twenties, was on a quest on what to learn from all his pain. Stephen Colbert, who also was struck with family tragedy—was a guest on one of his episodes. Stephen's father and two brothers were killed in a plane crash when Stephen was only ten years old. Cooper brought up a quote he'd read in another interview with Colbert: "If you're grateful for your life, then you have to be grateful for all of it."

Cooper asks him, "How can you be grateful for the death of somebody you've loved, or how can you be grateful for a terrible loss that you've experienced?"

"I haven't the slightest idea. I just know the value of it. I lost my father and my brothers, Peter and Paul, when I was ten. And that realization did not come until I was on the doorstep of middle age. Literally walking down the street, I was struck with this realization that I had a gratitude for the pain of that grief. It doesn't take the pain away. It doesn't make the grief less profound in some ways. It makes it more profound because it allows you to look at it. It allows you to examine your grief in a way that it is not, like holding up a red hot ember in your hands, but rather seeing that pain as something that can warm you and light your knowledge of what other people might be going through. Which is really just another way of saying there is a value to having experienced it."[9]

That story really resonated with me, in particular, because I could never figure out why I didn't feel like celebrating on my alive day (the day I was injured, April 12, 2012). We recalibrated soldiers called it "alive day" as if it were a day of honor, like a birthday. I've never felt that way, but more than ten years in, hearing this perspective helped me reshape how I saw it and now be grateful for it. I finally saw my alive day as a day of reflection on what's happened and how far we've come since my wife got that phone call. For hours she wouldn't know if I was going to live or die. I realized how grateful I am to celebrate because those injuries should've ended my life. Had I only focused on the negative, I wouldn't be able to appreciate all that has happened since.

It is not just the loss of a loved one or the threat of losing your own life that can be seen in a new light; it can be anything—like the loss of a job. Robert, whom you met in a previous chapter, had been at a growing nonprofit in Chicago for several months when he was fired. He could have been mad, bitter, spiteful, blaming his boss for setting himself up to fail; instead he looked at it as a learning opportunity. He was grateful that he took a minute and knew when to bend the knee. He ate a whole lot of humble pie and parlayed it into work on probation for the company to show that he could do indeed to the job, and four months later, they reinstated him. He turned around what could have been a massive blow to his ego and finances (he was in process of buying a house with a kid on the way, talk about stress) to see a great opportunity to prove himself. He chose the long game to see it through. He was grateful to have the presence of mind to do that. And he was grateful for the challenge because what he pulled off in the face of that challenge was quite a feat. He showed that we shouldn't ever plateau as a human being, and to be grateful for moments that make us step up.

Not everyone needs something as grand as an alive day to remind them to be grateful for what they have. Here are a few ways to cultivate this into your life.

Write Down Just One Thing…Maybe Five

The pen is mightier than the sword, the saying goes, and in the case of helping improve our mood and outlook, this is doubly true. Writing down what you are grateful for is a great way to get started. And I stress writing it down rather than just saying it out loud—the physical act of writing increases its effectiveness simply because we remember it better. For James, it was as small as writing down one thing. One thing, once a day, for twenty-one days. "If you just wake up every morning and write one thing that you're grateful for down on a piece of paper for twenty-one days, six months later, you will still reap the benefits: less anxiety. Just be happier. Before I practiced this, I was a negative Nancy. Say I won the lottery. I would want all the money in the denomination of fives. I wouldn't take the money unless it was all in fives, meaning I could never see the good in anything; rather, I would only see the imperfections. I would only concentrate on what was wrong. But now I'm that overly happy asshole that everyone hates. It was super hard to begin with, but eventually you trick your brain into doing so the next day and the next. It became a game to spend all day looking for three things I'm grateful for." There are impressive studies that show the act of expressing gratitude—in writing—improves mood and overall happiness. And the more they wrote, the more gratitude they felt.[10]

When should you do it? There is not universal consensus, so I suggest that you just get started. Try to do it twice or three times a week and see if you can go daily. What time of day, you ask? Morning? Night? Again the jury is out—so, much like exercise, do it when you will most likely keep it consistent.

Do it diligently. It comes back to having a choice. Make that choice that every morning when you wake up you will write down three things you're grateful for. Or maybe at the end of the day, you write three things that happened that day that were positive. And don't stress if something seems too small for thanks (a hot cup of coffee! No traffic!)—the simple maneuvering from negative to positive is what is important.

For Ray, "Practicing gratitude was a game changer because I used to wake up and I'd be pissed off and feeling sorry for myself. I couldn't see what was in front of me. In the army, I had seen every freaking shitshow overseas and lived in squalid conditions in training and while deployed for combat operations. But I couldn't appreciate that I have a house. I had running water. I have a beautiful wife—married thirty-five years. Once I started practicing gratitude, I started to realize all the things that I had, but it took me that practice... I couldn't see what was in front of me because I was stuck in my own head. Or I would only see what other people had. Social media is terrible for that, with everyone posting and boasting their best version of themselves. And with my repression of emotions, it was like say saying cake tastes delicious and not having the sense of taste. Initiating gratitude was excruciatingly hard as I had swallowed so much of my feelings for so long. But once I stopped hiding my feelings, I started experiencing and appreciating the present, the here and now. Since I experienced a lot of loss and the battlefield, I just used to say I was happy to be alive—but now I can say that I know why I am here and I am to be HERE."

It will take some work. And regular practice. It can be as simple as noticing a fantastic sunset or a morning walk on a beach. That fluffermuffin of a dog who greets you with unconditional love every morning. It'll help you stop and take a good look around to appreciate those things, and believe me, the more often you do this, the more you will see what to be grateful for.

Show Appreciation

When my son was born, we named him Dax. Nope, it's not a family name, but the combination of the names of the two medics that saved my life on that fateful day in April 2012. After the bomb blasted me in the air and then gravity plunged me back onto the hard dirt, I lay like a turtle on my back, with my right arm and leg gone, left leg still dangling, barely hanging on. Medics Dan Bateson and Alexander Voyce came running over to work on me.

"Don't worry about you're not going to save me…go save my guys," I managed to eke out, but they ignored me as they worked together to place tourniquets on all of my limbs and get an IV into me, all the while assuring me I was going to make it. Fast-forward about a five years later, when our son was born. It didn't take too long for us to come up with a name. It was Kelsey who suggested it. "What about Dax? What about taking the D and the A and the X from both the names and putting them together?" I loved the idea. What an honor to be able to name my son after the two men who saved my life.

Now, you don't have to go renaming your kids to show your appreciation or gratitude for those who helped you; a simple "I appreciate you" or "thank you" will go a long way.

Think Positively, Even When Negativity Creeps In

I am not going to lie and tell you that ever since practicing gratitude, I now never think back and wonder how life could have been, or that I don't let the little life's annoyances bother me. Nope, negative thoughts still creep in, and even though gratitude is a great buffer, sometimes I let those thoughts get to me. I may be in the shower and start thinking, *Man, how the hell is this my life? How are my arms and legs just gone? This is not going the way that I had my life planned out.* But then, I make a conscious effort to replace that negative thinking with positive thoughts. Immediately, I volley three positive thoughts to counteract the three negatives: I have wonderful kids, a great wife, a great career. Cut off that negativity at its knees.

Gratitude Chasing

Can you think of anything that brings you joy? Here are several ways to turn that gratitude switch on:

Writing thank-you notes

Volunteer work

Acts of kindness

Journaling

Exercising

Dance party!

Taking a walk—preferably in nature

Listening to music

Watching/reading something uplifting

The practice of gratitude, when done right and regularly, can profoundly change your resilience game—both mentally and physically. And one thing that should always be on your thank-you list is your friends and family. In fact, studies that show that a regular gratitude practice benefits social relationships across the board[11]—family, friends, coworkers, neighbors, even strangers. And there is nothing like a support system that carries you into the light when you are in the darkest corners of your mind. Let's give them some love, shall we?

PRINCIPLE #7

Get a Battle Buddy

Never Underestimate the Power of a Support System

When I first got injured, I suffered in silence—I didn't want anyone to know that I was in pain or hurting. As I mentioned earlier, the military preferred a stiff upper lip; talking about feelings was a sign of weakness. So, I never talked to a medical practitioner about how I felt when I got injured. It's not the preferred method, but that's how I am wired.

Looking back, I know that isn't the best course of action, but fortunately I was one of the lucky ones who had an amazing family to lean on as well as fellow rehabilitated (or what I like to call recalibrated) soldiers to talk to, which felt very cathartic. Accepting help is very humbling and can be one of the hardest pills people will have to swallow after any trauma. I gradually understood that having that support system—and opening up to that support system—made all the difference. It also gave me the motivation to push forward.

I do a lot of speaking engagements, and out on the road I encounter thousands of people from all walks of life who come to hear me speak. One common denominator of the people who come up to me after a speech is that they feel alone in their own struggles. What do I tell them? We have to realize that while our individual experiences may differ, the struggle is the same. Ninety-nine point nine percent of all human beings struggle. It's just what we do. Seek out that support system you need to get you through. Finding people who are going through the same thing will take away that loneliness and hopelessness. You need those close to you as you battle your trauma (as you'd do for them). *Resilience* is partly *reliance* on that support system. Liz, whom you met in the "Principle #1" chapter, knows that well. After her daughter Colleen died, she relied on her best friend, Karen. "Unwavering, she carried all of the anger that I couldn't carry. She was the one who would swear every curse word and then make up some when I couldn't." Having Karen being so supportive was integral in Liz being able to get through the excruciating pain, expletives and all.

There is a saying in the military: "Got your six." It means, "I got your back." As you probably know, the military is a fan of using the hours of the clock in many instances (like military time), and such is the case in strategizing positions. If an individual is moving in the twelve o'clock position, the six o'clock position would be in the rear. Hence, "Got your six" meant that that person was watching out for an enemy attacking from behind. This is what your circle of friends and family should be for you—and you for them.

CONNECTION IS CRUCIAL

We are by nature social beings, and so having meaningful connection throughout our lives is crucial to our well-being. A Harvard study—apparently the longest study on human behavior—has found that people who have deep personal relationships with others are overwhelmingly happier than people who don't.[1] Translation? You could be a billionaire and have all the material things you want in life and still be miserable. Money will not bring you happiness; status will not bring you happiness; having deep personal connections will. It does not just affect emotional health; it also affects your physical health. One recent study found that seniors who consider themselves lonely have a 59 percent higher risk of physical and mental health decline and a 45 percent greater risk of death.[2] Other studies liken loneliness to smoking fifteen cigarettes a day.[3] Yikes.

And it's not quantity, it's quality. You may have more than a thousand friends on Facebook, but do you have someone that you can actually sit down with and have a conversation about anything meaningful, beyond talking about the latest football playoff games or the latest celebrity breakup? While it is fun to talk pop culture, having someone to confide in when a more serious or consequential issue comes up will play a big role in how you are able to bounce back. Having someone to lean on has been shown to relieve stress and markedly improve your resilience as a result.[4]

And it has also been shown that connection is even more important to those who have gone through hardship.[5] Just like the guys I wanted to be in my foxhole on the front lines, you want a support system that will help you get through anything. You need people close to you to lean on as you battle whatever is in life (as you'd do the same for them). No person is an island, as they say, and I know that from hard-won experience. As mentioned earlier, in the unwritten rulebook of the military, we like to say, "Shit rolls downhill." That can mean passing off more mundane (and frankly shitty, pun intended) tasks to lower ranks. But it also means not letting your rank and file know about anything personal you may be going through, and that's why I never talked to anybody at first about how I was feeling. But I knew, deep down, I needed not only to open up about how I felt, but also to accept help, which was very humbling and can be one of the hardest pills that people will have to swallow after trauma or injury. I gradually understood that having that support system—and opening up to that support system—made all the difference. It also gave me the motivation to continue on.

It will be easier and more beneficial if that support system is already set in place and is there when you need it. My pal Mike, whom you met in the "Principle #2" chapter, had a ready safety net when he lost everything in the fire.

"My phone was just blowing up off the hook. It got to a point where I actually had to shut my phone off, just so I could try and figure out things. My office gave me the time off I needed, and my insurance company had gotten me a hotel within hours. But my wallet didn't make it out of the fire, and all I had on was a pair of boxers. Luckily, I had my gym bag and pair of shoes in my truck. A bit later, a rep that I worked with called me up and said, 'I heard you're having a rough day.'

"I said, 'Yes. You know, that's kind of an understatement.'

"'Hey, why don't you meet me at Mills Fleet Farm at four p.m.,' referring to the local goods store. So, I did. And we went inside and walked around. The next thing you know, he asked me, 'What size pants you wear?'

"Before I could protest, he just started throwing clothes and necessities in a cart. The next day, I found out a close friend of mine had started a GoFundMe page, and by the end of the week, it had close to $20,000 in it. I was embarrassed, but he told me, 'I want you to look at this and I want you to look at the people that care for you.' And while it felt weird and awkward to take it—I had never needed charity before—it showed me how much love and support I had around me, and that carried me for months."

Don't Isolate

Trauma survivors may have trouble connecting with their close family members or friends. The symptoms of PTSD can "cause problems with trust, communication, and closeness, which impact the way they interact with others."[6] You may feel hesitant to reach out for fear of being judged, or out of pride. If this is a behavior you are falling into, figure out your own way to bring back people in your life. You may be struggling with an act as simple as getting out of bed in the morning—and a call to a friend just may be the antidote for it.

Ask for Help When Needed...

Before the injury, I used to be able to bear-hug a washing machine when moving and follow it up with the dryer. But then, I got my arms and legs taken away, and I needed help. It can feel like a HUGE burden to feel "helpless" after being so independent, but you need to get over that. Rather, feel so fortunate to have people who love you who can help; for me, it was giving me water, feeding me, and just providing love and emotional support. They are good at things that I'm not very good at. For instance, they are really good at putting my legs on. I don't trust a lot of people to do it, either, because it's really weird. But I can honestly say my dad, my father-in-law, and my wife have been the beneficiaries of seeing me in my underpants. I also enlisted my buddy Zach once, when we were on a business trip in Florida. One morning, I had asked him to be at the ready to toss me a towel when I got out of the shower.

But as I was lathering up, I started thinking, "I'm gonna do it by myself. I'm Mr. Independent." So, instead of calling for him when I was done, I tried to step out of the shower on my own, but my leg slipped out from underneath me. BAM! I fell hard on the cold hard tile. I had to crawl across the floor out of the bathroom to get to the bed. My legs were still in the shower. It looked like a whole bomb went off again. Zach came in, his mouth agape, looking at the aftermath. "What happened here?"

"Oh, man, why'd you leave me?" I joked, deflecting blame onto him. If I had just waited and had him help me out, my butt cheeks would not have been swollen and bruised purple like a ripe plum for weeks. Lesson learned.

But Don't Overdo It

Don't have so much pride that you don't ask for help if you need it (like me), but also understand that asking too many times is not doing yourself any favors. So, just find that balance. You want to rely on people, but you don't want to be so dependent on them that you can't do anything for yourself—make sense?

During my recovery process, there was a fine line between "Can I do it?" and "Do I *want* to do it?" And it took a little bit of tough love on my wife's or my parents' part. Take my dad. He would often come with me to a physical therapy session. There'd he be, off to the side, encouraging me. "Hey, man, come on, pick it up. You can do this." I'd be sitting there, thinking, *Do you wanna come here and do it yourself? Stop pushing me.* But at the end of the day, he knew I could give a bit more effort, which meant I would recover faster. As much as I hated being told to do something, I knew they were pushing me to do something so I could get better.

AND THEY WILL PUSH YOU

Enock Glidden was born in 1978 with spina bifida, an often debilitating condition in which the spine and spinal cord do not grow properly. Growing up in a small town in northern Maine, he was the only kid in a wheelchair for miles around, and so everybody knew him. "That meant I had a really huge group of people who were basically willing to help me anytime I wanted to try something. My parents also always told me I could do anything, and so that really gave me a leg up (no pun intended). So, whenever I get an idea to do something, there was always someone there. I had a phys ed teacher, Bob Dyer, in junior high. On the first day we met, he walked up to me and asked me if I could do twenty push-ups in my wheelchair. I replied, 'Well, no, I can do forty.' And I don't think I'd ever done forty push-ups to that point in my life, but I pulled it off. From that day on, he never treated me differently—in fact, he pushed me to try new things. And even when we were playing soccer in phys ed class, he would make me join in and let me hold the ball; he always found ways for me to do things other kids were doing."

Dyer encouraged him to join the basketball team, took him hunting, and eventually got him into wheelchair racing. He completed the Maine marathon a few times in high school and, later, started climbing. He found a wonderful adaptive sports organization called Paradox Sports, and that is where his climbing journey really took off. What first started out as small climbs in New York and New Hampshire climbs turned into Yosemite Park's El Capitan's 3000 in 2020...and he hopes to climb Washington's Mt. Rainier in the future. His teacher taught him not to say "How I can't," but instead ask "How can I?" and he is now showing others how to, by serving as an ambassador for Paradox Sports.

Don't Forget the Trauma-Adjacent

It is understood in the military that the burden of sacrifice is not only a sacrifice for the service member, but also for the spouse and children, who need a special kind of resilience. It doesn't seem to matter if they came along before, during, or after injury and time in service. These kids endure countless moves, leaving friends and new schools, doctor's appointments and new normals, temporary housing, and waiting rooms, yet they don't know any different. Your family is incredibly strong and brave as they support their loved one—they are warriors in their own right. And they also are affected by it: A 2010 St. Louis University study showed how people who simply observed or witnessed the stress of others also became stressed.[7] Since the observers' cortisol levels spiked as well, the study concluded that stress can spread like a contagion, meaning that you could "catch" the emotion, much like you would a cold.[8] So, they, too, need love and support in these times.

My wife, Kelsey, the trouper she is, found her do-or-die support group early on at Walter Reed. Apparently, they had gotten labeled the "Walter Reed clique" soon after she and a few other women—all wives of amputee soldiers—had all bumped into one another in the hospital's break room late at night. Jenn, one of the wives, was constantly at the bedside of her husband, Drew, who had just been beginning his military career when he was injured in Afghanistan. She was pregnant with her first child when he got injured on May 12, 2012, a month after me. He had been deployed for only three weeks. His right leg had to be amputated; his left was salvaged, but it had sustained 60 percent muscle loss. It was touch and go for a while. "We were in triage mode at that point. All of our partners had been injured around the same time, but none of each knew each other. And it's not like I went into the hospital and I saw Kelsey and said, 'Oh, hey, can we be friends?' No, we met in the ice room at night. It was where everybody all filled her husband's water bottles at night like clockwork. Our husbands always wanted cold water. And we just fell into each other's paths. We might have been a crying shoulder one night, or just a needed break from the constant care of another. We'd start to intentionally sneak out of our husbands' rooms and head to the break room, hoping we would bump into each other. It took only a few weeks to form a bond that lasts to this day. It felt as if something bigger chose us, because we didn't choose each other. Our paths crossed for a reason."

It's a Two-Way Street

Giving support is just as important as receiving it. Research shows that, as Dr. Neff has stated, the more supported we feel, the more resilient we feel. And guess what, the same is true when we give support to others. It makes us more resilient too. Giving support is just as good as receiving it.

What do I mean by this? Support swings in both directions. That's the power of the support system—that constant straddle between that mentor-mentee relationship; you're both learning from each other as you lean on and challenge each other, but at different times. It's like Todd Nicely, who helped me get out of that funk when I first arrived at Walter Reed. At times, I would be his anchor when he was going through a rough patch. And at other times, those roles can be reversed as you help somebody who's trying to avoid the same scars or learn the same lessons that you did.

And you don't have to wait to be in a jam to get this benefit. Be aware. Is someone around you needing help now? Robert likes to remind himself of all the help he had along the way.

"I was blessed in that I had the resources to be able to do this thing and take the risk I did. With all the variables in the air, I had so many people in my corner, too, in the form of my wife, especially, and my friends. I wish I could say we lived in a world where more people had that, because there are many people who don't. They don't have the ability to even make the choice."

What he means is that the media and public often praise people who had "a profile in courage" and rose up despite the odds. We all love a by-the-bootstraps Horatio Alger story, but we tend to forget that his protagonists often had benefactors that helped along the way. There are many who aren't so lucky. We'll talk about this more in the "Principle #11" chapter, but why not help someone who needs a bit of wind beneath their wings?

Robert continues: "I care to live in a world where more people have that, quote, unquote, rich uncle or something like that to afford them the space and the grace to be able to come into their full selves. Not all of us have that. In the American experience, where we live in a culture that so values rugged individualism, whether we realize it or not, it's almost like we lionize people so much and remove aspects of their story where they received help from someone else, as though they did this all on their own. I wouldn't be where I am right now without somebody in my corner who had my back." He knows the power of that support—and he continues today to do what he can to be that person in the corner for someone else.

Reaching Out

Sometimes we feel that our friends and family may not "get" what we are going through. Support can come in many forms. If you feel that you need outside help, here are a couple of ways to go about it.

1. Reach out to someone you know who is going through or has gone through a similar process. Whether it's getting a divorce, losing a partner or child, being laid off, or coming home from active deployment—talking to someone who has walked in your footsteps can offer you just the right insight and support to help you get through. And that person will most likely appreciate it, as they will feel they have helped pay it forward, as they, too, probably had someone help them through.

2. Talk to a therapist. If you feel overly anxious, angry, or are thinking harmful thoughts, it is time to bring in the professionals. Some feel going to a therapist shows "weakness," but it shows a lot of strength to know you need help. There are also great therapy groups that can help keep you on the right path, from

bereavement groups to Al-Anon and AA. (Please note that while online therapy groups can be effective, do your research and ensure they are HIPAA compliant.)

Whether it's your family, cubicle mates, strangers in the hospital break room, or your gym teacher, having a supportive group of people cheering you on is essential to helping you build resilience (as you build theirs). And you'll need that ongoing connection as you move forward, because you can't quit now.

Never Give Up, Never Quit, Ever

Push Yourself Past Your Own Personal Best

Perseverance runs through the Mills family blood. Growing up in the small town of Vassar, Michigan, you needed it. Like so many of our neighbors, we had a 20-acre hobby farm, and so at an early age, I learned to weed, hoe, cut wood, and clean out the barn—I learned to do anything and everything that had to do with running a farm. We were spared a lot during the school year, but every summer morning between six thirty and seven, my dad would wake us up to weed his garden out back or pick what was ripe and ready, like his tomatoes, corn, squash, and cucumbers. Let me tell you, that "garden" was the size of a damn football field. "Dig this hole, build that trench, cut this grass, or weed these two rows...," whatever he needed us to do that day, we did it, usually under the brutally steamy August sun. But this was my dad; he always worked his ass off; he was a truck driver and maintenance engineer when he wasn't busy on the farm, and my mom, who started working at the age of thirteen, had a steady job at the pickle factory. We were taught by example that life is hard work and to keep going until the job's done—and the job was never done.

So, it was ingrained in me that you worked hard—no ifs, ands, or buts—and always keep doing something to improve. I brought all that into my sports—karate, basketball, football—I always seemed to be playing something. I practiced hard, always striving to be better. Giving up or quitting at something just wasn't in our DNA. Then I joined the military, whose entire philosophy is "Never quit." It could be a matter of life or death.

It wasn't until that fateful April day in 2012 that I came to consider giving up. The shock of the newness of my situation didn't allow me to see a way out of it.

Those first days of my injury shook me to the core—there was no knowing if I would ever be strong enough to support my family again. Those days were tough for everybody. I went from a strong, able-bodied staff sergeant fighting on the front lines to waking up to my mom wiping my butt or my wife feeding me. I certainly didn't want to be a burden to anyone, and I didn't want to let anyone down. If there was ever a time I felt like quitting, it was then. When I had the chance, I even gave Kelsey an out. I told her she didn't sign up for this, married to someone who couldn't feed himself. (I like to joke that she stuck with me, if only for the handicapped parking.) But eventually, I saw that I had a choice between two options—do or don't. To lie there and never get out of that bed, or persevere and push on. It may be that I was a military man through and through, and that kind of training gave me a tough, "do or die trying" mindset. I decided I would not spend the rest of my life living in the past—that was not how I wanted to be for my wife, kids, or other vets. It took me time to figure out my new normal, and it meant remembering how I was brought up, and that was never to give up. Instead, I had the mindset of "I dare you to tell me that I can't do this."

It was probably two weeks into my recovery. I was doing sit-ups, and the occupational therapist asked, "Do you want to take a break?"

I responded, "No, I'm not going to stop. I'm never going to quit."

"Well, I guess that was a silly question."

Yup, it was. And that is where my motto famously was born. I said that I'd never give up and I'll never quit, and it stuck. If you are reading this book, I know you don't want to give up; you are looking for ways to move on, press ahead. So I am here to tell you—I am living proof to never give up. Go on, push through.

And I am not talking about hitting your head against the wall for no good reason, or in my case, trying to imagine my arms and legs miraculously growing back. You can't force something to happen that ain't going to happen. Grit, perseverance, persistence, whatever you want to call it, is about adapting to your situation. Okay, so you hit some headwinds. How do you adjust the sails to keep going forward? I live by the "Never give up, never quit" motto because I know if I get knocked down, if I fall, it's not easy for me to get up. My kids won't see me just fall; they'll see me flip over on my knees and put my arm on something to brace so I can stand back up. It may not be how other fathers get up, but I am still showing them that it's not whether you got knocked down; it's whether you get up (famously coined by the legendary football coach Vince Lombardi). And in my case, it is about adapting. Doing the same thing over and over again only to fail is not persistence; that is just being stubborn. Persistence is looking at the situation and how you handle it—if it is not working, what would work? All this is to say that grit is about always trying your best, but also learning and adapting.

DO YOUR BEST, EVEN IF IT'S SECOND BEST

As I have said before, a lot of what goes into resilience is changing your attitude. One of the tweaks I've made in my own life is that winning isn't everything (well, not true, but you can't win all the time). Second best is always a reminder that you can never be perfect. Coming in second, in fact, is okay if you gave it your all. I am not saying *not* to try to get that top podium; on the contrary: I put all my energy into trying every day to be my best self. That's when you really start to succeed, by pushing yourself past your own personal bests.

Case in point: My daughter, Chloe, had a meet where she didn't do as well as she wanted for gymnastics. After the meet, she came up to me a little bit teary-eyed.

"Chloe," I consoled her as we drove home, "I can remember sitting in that same passenger seat, with my dad in the driver's seat, telling him how upset I was that I lost at a wrestling match. That I didn't do my best and I didn't win. The truth is, you learn the most about yourself right now. You've got to pick your head up because you at least competed. You showed up, and you tried your best." After a few moments, I added, "Do you want to quit?"

Luckily, she replied, "No! I'll just keep doing what Dory does. 'When life gets you down, you know what you got to do? Just keep swimming, swimming, swimming…,'" taking a line out of one of our favorite animated movies, *Finding Nemo*. That's my girl.

Not everything is going to be a win, but you keep pushing. "Charlie Mike" is the military code for "Continue Mission"—pushing through adversity no matter the difficulties. No matter what you set out to do in life, you are going to get crushed by somebody, but you can get up off the ground while you're hurting, and that extra effort—the never give up, never quit attitude—will propel you to the top. Continue the mission, no matter what.

AND WHEN MORE SETBACKS HAPPEN...

By now, you know that nothing in life is guaranteed, and often things come along that knock us off our course. Whatever happened, we can't go back and change it. We can't hide it. We can't bury the problem, as it will only get bigger with time. So, once you acknowledge it, a good practice to help you determine your next steps is to give yourself some perspective. Best-selling author and everyone's wannabe dinner guest Brené Brown has a great way to look at the nature of setbacks: "Will this issue be a big deal in five minutes? Five hours? Five days? Five months? Five years?"[1] What is your answer? If the setback is temporary and won't matter much in time, don't let it get in your way. If it does, then the only way to get over a setback is through it. So much about grit and persistence is not so much doing something ad nauseam, even if it isn't working; it is the knowledge that it isn't working and the resolve to change course. So much is about understanding something isn't for you, and you need to move on. Grit helps see what you are capable of.

Pam Swan knows all too well what she is capable of. I know Pam from working with actor Gary Sinise and his foundation, where she is vice president of military relations and business development for Veterans United Home Loans. A nationally recognized expert on military personal finance, she grew up poor. Pam was the fifth child of six; her mother had her first child at the age of thirteen and the sixth (who died at three months old) at nineteen.

"My family had been living in a junkyard where my dad worked in a small town, Milford, Illinois. Population: 1,700 people. By the time I was born, my dad was working for a farmer, and we had moved into what is called a brooder house—in essence, an octagon-shaped chicken coop. Sheetrock was put in to create two makeshift walls that helped divide the structure into 'rooms.' There wasn't a toilet nor was there a tub, but that didn't really matter since we didn't have any running water anyway. Our grandmother lived close by, so sometimes we would be able to bathe there. Otherwise, I used baby powder as a DIY substitute to put in my hair to soak up the grease and dirt. Life was about survival. All the kids shared a double bed, with the three boys sleeping at the head, and me and my sister sleeping at the foot of the bed. When I got a little older, I raked leaves or babysat so I could buy clothes to look presentable at school. I knew we weren't 'normal.'

"The coop was so dilapidated that it flooded too much for even my father; in time, he managed to scrape enough money together for us to rent a two-bedroom mobile home—we thought we were kings and queens! While our home environment was nominally better, home life wasn't any better. My parents fought all the time, always on the verge of getting a divorce; at the age of thirteen, I decided to run away with one of my brothers. We did so by hotwiring cars (something my brother knew how to do) to get us to one place and then stealing another, crisscrossing towns as we headed south. We made it all the way to Arkansas, sleeping underneath the overpasses; we'd sleep under 'blankets' made of tall weeds we had pulled, and burn what we could for heat. After a few weeks, the police caught up to us, and they brought us home. Charges were brought for stealing the first car, and I had to move back in with my parents until the hearing. Unfortunately, they didn't seem to care how we were doing or why we ran away—they only hoped the whole ordeal 'taught us a lesson.'

"When our case came up, we told the judge all that happened—about how we were raised and how we felt it was our only chance to get out. After listening to our defense, the judge concluded: 'If I had any way to change this sentence to give it to the parents, I would. Your time has been served.' And I remember thinking that that was the first confirmation from anybody that my life was not normal.

"Afterward, my parents looked at me and said, 'If you're going to run away again, then just leave now.' And so I did. I walked away. I started working at odd jobs: a coffee shop, a laundry room at a nursing home, wherever who would hire a thirteen-year-old. I rented a room from a woman who lived close to my high school. I dropped out of school, though, when I was a sophomore, and went to work full-time. At the age of eighteen, I was living on my own and managing a couple of different restaurants. I relished paying my bills—on time. I could flush my toilet without having to use a bucket. And I never begrudged going to work and leaving school. I was able to contribute to the community and to myself."

In a few years, Pam would meet her husband, who was in the army. They married and moved to where he was stationed at Fort Campbell, Kentucky, then later Fort Bliss, Texas. She took classes here and there, and then she took a course that certified her as a financial counselor and planner. Now, she puts that to use to help veterans. Her story is a remarkable one of resilience and an extreme case of never quitting. "When I put my head on my pillow at night, I need to feel proud knowing that I did some good in the world. If I can do that, I had a good day."

With everything stacked against her, Pam's stick-to-it-ness helped her rise above what was indeed a traumatic childhood—one that no one should ever have to endure. Somehow, she had the wherewithal to take a long-term view, focusing on what she could control. She always seemed to find a reason to keep going, even if it was simply to have accomplished a good hard day's work. Your story of persistence may not be so dire, but the idea behind never giving up is the same: If you stick to a deliberate approach, making small changes or improvements, step by step, day by day, moment by moment, you'll soon find that you've made significant progress. When you feel that you don't have any more to give, remember you do. Take a deep breath, push through.

Somehow Pam found agency, despite the odds. Agency is the opposite of helplessness; instead of caving to what life had handed her, she was able to rise above and take responsibility in creating her own future. She knew her choices were limited, but she had the capacity to be able to choose the best out of the lot. No matter your situation, the feeling that you are in control of what happens, no matter the circumstance, is a very profound and empowering feeling.

IT'S ALL ABOUT HAVING A GROWTH MINDSET

Pam is a perfect example of someone having grit. Psychologist Angela Lee Duckworth, the best-selling author of *Grit: The Power of Passion and Perseverance*, defines grit as "perseverance and passion for long-term goals." In her words:

"Grit entails working strenuously toward challenges, maintaining effort and interest over the years despite failure, adversity, and plateaus in progress."[2] People are born with various levels of grit, but Duckworth contends that it is a trait that develops through experience. One key to improving it, as she points out in her TED Talk, is by shifting your mindset from a fixed to a growth orientation.

Tips on Helping You Stick It Out

1. **Don't overthink it.** Ah, the burden of large brains—just more room to ruminate and second-guess everything. But try not to obsess about how far you have to go, and what challenges you have to face in order to get things back on track. You'll soon find that you've made considerable progress. You never want to become too overwhelmed with the work yet to come. Stick to a deliberate approach and have a setbacks-will-come-but they-won't-break-me attitude to keep you going.

2. **Take your time.** Remember, there are no shortcuts. And that is okay. Whether it is getting over a death or trying to write a book (ahem), anything successful takes hard work, constant focus, diligence, and effort.

3. **Always be curious.** If you are reading this book, my guess is that you may have already tried therapy. You may or may not have found it helpful. If not, don't let that dissuade you from looking for answers elsewhere. You can do your own research, listen to a podcast, or go to a lecture that can help you on your journey toward growth. Who knows, one author or personality may write (or say) precisely the right thing you needed to read (or hear) at that time that helps you change your perspective. Being curious will help you find answers in unexpected places.

4. **Be a one-percenter.** The 1 percent rule is the theory of making tiny changes that add up. A series of small achievable improvements is easier to manage than trying to tackle a big one all at once. This will help you stay on course. Take one day at a time, even one hour at a time if you have to.

5. **Be careful about perfectionism.** High achievers, watch out: you tend to be much harder on yourself and really go overboard in terms of never quitting. Growth can be a long, hard road, and sometimes progress can be slow. Be patient. Give yourself enough credit. External goals won't necessarily help you achieve fulfillment. Think about what really matters and concentrate on that.

The theory behind this idea of fixed and growth mindsets was conceived by psychologist Carol Dweck, which is laid out in her brilliant work *Mindset*. In it, she shows how success in school, work, and nearly every aspect of our lives can be dramatically influenced by how we think about our talents and abilities. People with a *fixed mindset*—those who believe that abilities are absolute—are less likely to flourish than those who believe that abilities can be developed (growth mindset). In other words, with a growth mindset, you see challenges as learning opportunities rather than as obstacles to overcome. Say you got fired…well, that really sucks, first of all. With a fixed mindset, you may view your situation as "All is lost." How will you possibly get another job? How are you going to support yourself or your family? With a growth mindset, you will see that with the freedom from a job (that you didn't like anyway), you have the time to think about what is next and find something that is more satisfying to you. Of course, you still have the stress of financial strain and an unknowable future, but once you see that your mindset is pliable, a whole world of opportunity and optimism shows up. Once we see these forces that hold us back, we have to make an active choice to shift our mindset. Because our mindset drives our behavior and the choices we make. Sometimes trauma can mess with that mindset, but that is where post-traumatic growth principles can help.

One of those things that can mess with that optimistic mindset is fear. Let's tackle that next.

Swim with the Sharks, Walk with the Horses

Make Fear Your Friend

Until recently, I had a textbook fear of sharks. I know, I know: I have parachuted out of planes, been trained to kill, and led dangerous missions to uncover land mines (we know how the last one turned out). I took on fear every day of the workweek. But truth be told, I had always been scared of a fish with a fin on it. And I am not sure where this fear came from, since sharks have never snuck into a Maine lake, as far as I know.

But not all fear is the same. The fear of sharks, heights, spiders—whatever makes your body recoil—is real, but there are much starker and debilitating fears that can take hold of us and stop us in our tracks. The fear of the unknown. The fear of failure. The fear of rejection. The fear of what other people think of you. The fear of the past repeating itself. When we struggle with something, fear is almost always a major factor in how we handle the struggle. In a bad marriage? The fear of the future—*Will I ever love again?*—keeps many people from leaving a toxic relationship. Struggling at work with a bad boss? Fear of speaking up (or quitting) may keep you in an unhealthy environment.

For me, the fear of failure hits home. When I was growing up and playing a lot of competitive sports, I never ever wanted to fail, and I took that fear to my military days as it folded in nicely with the military's hard-ass philosophy of always having a game face. I always wanted to make sure that I led from the front and never showed any weakness, because if I did, my guys would lose faith in me. I knew that if that happened, they wouldn't follow my orders that were meant to keep them alive. That fear drove me.

When I became injured, I was confronted with a new, seemingly insurmountable fear. How the hell was I going to take care of my wife and daughter with no legs or arms? Who did I think I was? Because I was certainly no longer Staff Sergeant Mills, fearless leader of combat soldiers. I was instead lying in a bed, helpless, limbless, and jobless. That immediate fear I had in that hospital bed lasted for weeks, months, even. No one saw it, though. I wouldn't let them. I wouldn't let fear win. I probably didn't handle this perfectly, but in the military you're taught that if you stop moving forward, you die. So, even though I couldn't physically move forward, I knew I had to move on emotionally. I used the fear as a motivating factor to help me, but I know for most of us, getting over our fears isn't easy. Why is that?

Well, I didn't know either. I didn't pay attention to biology so much in high school. I was too busy mapping out my latest school prank. But when we were putting together our PATHH program at TMF, I got a primer on how we physiologically deal with fear. I found out that while none of us particularly likes to be afraid, we are hardwired to deal with it when it does come our way. We have a tiny, almond-shaped region in the brain called the amygdala that detects "Danger, Danger!" and kicks our hormones cortisol and adrenaline into high gear. Our heart begins to race; we may get a little short of breath; our pupils dilate. This is that flight-or-fight response we discussed in the "Principle #5" chapter, and this reaction was lifesaving back in the day when we had to run from, say, a lion that looked at us like we were its next meal. Our senses kicked in to save our butt. Today, we aren't usually in a situation where we have to react to a lethal, physical threat (unless we are on the battlefield or being chased down an alley), but our body does read other, less discernible stresses as threats. So, whether it is a looming deadline or bad highway traffic, or more serious and constant pressures like being in the throes of a divorce or a victim of emotional abuse, this primordial part of the brain screams, "SNAFU!" and our body goes into react mode. Eventually, after the perceived threat is gone, our hippocampus, our "thinking" area of the brain, kicks in. It further assesses the situation, and we start to think more rationally and may see things differently. Our brain feels first, thinks later.

Before I end the biology lesson, there's another interesting statistic that stuck with me when we were developing PATHH: we have eighty-six billion cells in the human brain, of which only a tiny portion is highly adaptable to new circumstances, or what the guys in the white coats call "cognitive flexibility."[1] While a small part of our cells can be flexible, the rest of them don't like change. For example, when something happens that you didn't expect, you can feel uneasy, stressed, right? It's because we have a natural affinity for certainty, for feeling safe and comfortable, and knowing what is going to happen next. We like routine. We like to be comfy. This is another factor that drives fear. Feeling safe and in control is the opposite of feeling fear. But as we all know, change is part of life—so fear is only natural.

Why am I telling you all this? It's for you to understand that fear is okay. To feel fear is natural and normal, but it is also the irrational, emotional side of you. And you can tackle it with the rational, perceptive, and thinking side of you. Some fear is good—it gets the blood going in the morning—but we need to be careful about how much is incoming, how severe, and how constant. It is that constant drum of unease and stress that can get us into trouble.

And the more you understand how your brain works, the easier it will be to understand yourself and tackle your fears… follow me? When I first found all this out, it made so much sense. Understanding what is going on is half the battle. I want you to see how fear can, in fact, be a major driving force in resilience, making us stronger than before. It is just how we look at it and decide what to do with that fear. Fear can limit us; it can let us be affected by what others say about us; ultimately, it can stop us from doing things we want to do in life, and in the case of resilience, prevent us from moving on, by avoiding the very issues that keep us stuck in the first place. For me and my fear of *Jaws*, I got myself to an aquarium and swam with the sharks (I was in a cage, but still). I am here to show you that it doesn't have to paralyze you—you can let it drive you.

There are a bunch of ways that fear can rear its ugly head. Sometimes the biggest fear we have is to show our true emotions and our vulnerabilities. While suppressing emotion can lead to a victory on the battlefield—no one wants a pal bawling his eyes out when you are about to engage the enemy—having this as your MO every day can become a problem. I have seen it with tons of military friends. They get to go home after a deployment to their wife or husband and are afraid to open up. They are afraid to talk about their experiences for fear that others will think less of them, that they are weak. And unfortunately, this can lead them to a host of issues down the road.

SEE A MAN ABOUT A HORSE

Resilience isn't about being unafraid. It's about knowing your fear and addressing it, and there is only one way to do that: head-on. Because if YOU can't get over a fear of something, how will you move past it? There is a popular saying about fear that is often quoted in the military: "The cave you fear to enter holds the treasure you seek." (You didn't think I had it in me to throw in some Joseph Campbell here, did you?) At the Travis Mills Foundation, we live by that quote, and we have made it our mission to teach its meaning to our guests, specifically in a therapy program that pairs veterans with horses. Yes, horses. Horses have been used in therapy for years because they are so attuned to human behavior. They are like a barometer—they can sense how you are feeling from 50 yards away. So, at the foundation retreats, we team up former soldiers who have trauma-related issues with horses to do one-on-one work. They spend some time with the animals, getting them to trust them and vice versa. The goal is to get the horse to trust the vet to lead. And he can't do that if he is scared. He has to exude confidence, not fear, to get the 800-pound animal to move. So, the vet has to shed the fear to be able to connect with the horse on an emotional level. Once that happens, we have them try to lead the horse. If the person keeps looking back to see if the horse is following them, the horse will start turning around or stop walking. It's the same thing that happens on patrol: if you are always turning around looking to make sure the guy behind you is doing what he's supposed to be doing, there is a lack of trust. You have to trust him, as he is trusting you to lead. So, as with the horse, if you turn around, he thinks that you're not confident. If you are confident, the horse will start following. It's something we hope they can take out of the foundation grounds and into their own life. If you can't get over a fear of something, how will you get that horse to believe in you? How will you get *yourself* to believe in you?

While I don't have the magic bullet on *how* you can do this—everyone is different—I can give you some tricks that I know have worked for me and others. It is often said that the opposite of fear is courage, and that speaks to my inner dude's "never quit" attitude. I just had to keep going. Iconic actor John Wayne said it way better than me: "Courage is being scared to death—but saddling up anyway."

SADDLE UP

While that may sound easier said than done, I am here to tell you that there are ways to push past that fear so you can finally move on. Otherwise, fear can take control of your life, if you let it. It can be a significant factor in any sort of decision-making (or the lack thereof) and, therefore, your happiness. So, here are several steps you can take to help you kick fear in the you-know-what:

1. Know what your fear is. Is there something in your life you want to change but don't? Knowledge is power.
2. Acknowledge that a bit of fear is good. It means it is taking you out of your comfort zone. Get comfortable with being uncomfortable.
3. Know that it is normal to feel this way, and many people feel fear. You are not alone.
4. Share your fear with others who will understand what you are going through.
5. Stop negative thinking in its tracks. When our mind wanders, it tends to go over to the dark side,[2] and that sort of negativity can lead to *more* negative thinking, like *I can't do it*, or *It will all go wrong*. Ask yourself, are these thoughts serving you? Or are they just messing with you?
6. Plan. Take it from the top brass—most of what the military does again and again is training and preparing; we saw action only a fraction of the time. Reducing uncertainty will make you feel more certain

things will work out. Sometimes, visualization can help. Think of a few scenarios and then visualize how each aspect would play out.

7. Call it. Realize that you have a choice—to get over the fear or not.

8. Give yourself a big "hooyah" for going for it. Be grateful for the strength you showed.

9. Debrief. Think about how you would improve— show a growth mindset. When I was in the 82nd Airborne, we'd review every mission. We called it AAR (after action review), and we'd dissect what happened and map out how we'd do better next time.

10. Repeat. What's next on your list of fears?

STOP DOIN' DONUTS

Let's talk about item 5, negative thinking, for a moment because I see so many people struggle with this. We touched on this a bit earlier in the book; it's what I call "doing donuts," because of all those thoughts going around and around in your head. *I'm not good enough. I am going to fail. No matter what I do, it will not be enough. It's too much. I can't do it.* Case in point: One of Kelsey's friends, Jenn, whom you met in the "Principle #7" chapter, was pregnant with her first child when her husband, Drew, got injured in Afghanistan on May 12, 2012, the day before Mother's Day. He had been deployed for only three weeks. His right leg had to be amputated; his left was salvaged, but it had sustained 60 percent muscle loss. Today, Jenn straddles between being a caretaker for Drew, who still has medical issues, and being a mom for her kids. She often feels overtaken by fear—fear that they can't give their kids a normal childhood. It is something she worries about every moment of every single day. But she has acknowledged her fear, confronts it head-on, and is grateful for pushing through. While she sees her only choice as being strong for her family, some days are harder than others. Here's a quick snapshot of her daily life:

"Last Halloween, I promised the kids that I would take them to the pumpkin patch. Drew was having a tough day physically, so I had to decide: does he go with us or do I let the kids down? I so wanted to give my kids that amazing childhood memory but at the same time, taking an amputee to a pumpkin patch has its own set of challenges. We decided to make the best of it. We had to bypass the wagon ride and clear paths along our walk to ensure there were no vines Drew could trip over, but that inconvenience outweighed our giving our kids the feeling we were like every other family.

"We may not be able to go on family bike rides the same way as our next-door neighbors can, but just because Drew can't do it doesn't mean that he doesn't enjoy watching. So, whenever I get overwhelmed or fearful, or feel like we aren't doing enough for our kids, I remind myself: I have the love of my life next to me. My son has his father. I have been blessed with my two other children. Our happiness may look different, but at the end of the day, it's still happiness."

See how Jenn turned around negative thoughts here? Quieting our own harshest critic is a tough one for a lot of people. Did you know that on a typical day, the brain averages six thousand thoughts,[3] and 80 percent of those are negative?[4] If you add to it a bad experience and the questioning that follows, I believe this number multiplies. That's a lot of crap swirling around up there. Worse, we cling to negative thoughts more than to positive ones. According to studies, negative experiences are easier to recall and in more detail because of how they affect us emotionally.[5] In boot camp, we'd often sing cadence as we did drills. I thought it was to keep us in step and alert, but now I know it was to help us focus, for sure, but also to help keep those shitty thoughts from creeping in.

Clear Your Head

Here are some quick, practical ways to help let go of those thoughts leaving dirt tracks in your head:

- **Just breathe, slowly.** We talked about this before, but this is important in settling the mind. This helps slow your heart rate by engaging the parasympathetic nervous system, which makes us feel calmer. Breathe in for 4, out for 4. My kids love this one.

- **Take a walk outside.** Walking in nature has been shown to lower our anxiety levels and also reduce blood pressure. So, get out there, make some tracks.
- **Meditate.** This can help calm our system down, and studies show it can even change how we process bad memories.[6] I don't do this myself, but I know many people who have found this to be incredibly helpful.
- **Listen to music.** Listening to soothing music (so maybe not the *Jaws* theme) is known to calm the central nervous system,[7] and triggers the release of our feel-good dopamine hormone.[8] Music can also help provide a distraction from stress[9] (much like what Kate Bush's "Running up that Hill" did for Max, shattering Vecna's mental hold on her in season 4 of *Stranger Things*).
- **Laugh.** This is my favorite, as anyone who knows me will tell you. I can't pass up a good joke. And in the military, humor was always a great deflection—whether it was to pass the time, boost morale, or defuse any intense situation. And it works—laughter has shown to help us take in more oxygen, release those feel-good endorphins that relax us, and lower those stress hormones. I've always joked that even though I lost both my legs and arm in the explosion, at least I didn't lose my humor.

WORK IT OUT

Our resilience is like a muscle. The more you practice facing your fears, the stronger you will be. The more we exercise our courage, the more we beat the fear, the better we'll get at it. The more challenges we give it, the more adaptable we'll be. The more experience we get, the better we'll be, the more perceptive we'll be. It's been shown that the more a person believes they can overcome their challenges, the more likely they are to do so.[10] Chloe Carmichael, PhD, psychologist and author of *Nervous Energy: Harness the Power of Your Anxiety*, posits that it is about control: When a person believes that they have the power to influence something, they are more inclined to manage it.[11] However, if they believe that things are out of control, then they will be less likely to be motivated.

It's the power of positive thinking, really, and by extension thinking in terms of the growth mindset versus the fixed mindset we talked about in the previous chapter. By thinking positively and imagining our success—rather than drowning in those self-defeating thoughts—we can reach new heights.

One way to do this is to switch up your negative thoughts and turn them into positive ones. Think you are never going to get ahead? Think instead how great it is going to feel when you get that corner office. Think you are doomed to be single because your last relationship went up in flames? Think how exciting it will be to meet someone new. Another technique when you are going down Negativity Road is thinking about what you would say if your best friend or sibling was going through the same thing. I bet you would give them a boatload of compassionate and positive advice. So, give yourself the same.

Trick Your Brain

If you need help in the power of positive thinking, turn on your TV and watch any sports game. Every game is a lesson in believing in yourself, because one team or one athlete always leaves the field the losing opponent. There is lots of failure happening. You can be the fittest competitor and athlete, but how well you trained and how fit you are is only half the battle. The mental part of the game, the psychology of performing, is the other half. At some point, you have to create some sort of mechanism that tricks your brain. Nomar Garciaparra, legendary shortstop for the Boston Red Sox and third baseman for the Cubs and Dodgers, had a whole ritual he would perform each time he stepped up to the plate, which involved a series of glove adjustments and toe-taps. He was using positive thinking to prepare himself for the next pitch. It was obvious that he was OCD about it, but it was to trick his brain into doing what he wanted: to focus and hit that ball when it whirled to him at 90 miles an hour. He was able to create a system that worked for him to make him be successful in his goals and banish the word "failure" from his mind.

UNDERSTAND THAT FEAR IS ALWAYS WITH US

And that is a good thing. It means we are doing something important, new, unfamiliar. It can also help us look at our trauma differently. Learn from it. Embrace it and realize that you looked fear right in its eyes and you were unbowed. It especially makes us look at death and grief differently. Remember Liz, who lost her husband in a car crash? She lost her daughter Colleen, also in a car accident, nearly thirteen years later.

"I used to be afraid of everything. Before my husband died, he used to joke, 'All you do is worry!' I would reply, 'I know, but think of all of the catastrophes we've averted because I worried about it!' And then he would say my chances of dying in an airplane crash are slim, and none. 'Far more likely, I'll be killed in a car crash.'

"Yeah, he said those words, which didn't mean a thing at the time. He continued, 'If your number's up, your number's up.' And now I agree with him. I used to be afraid of everything now and just kind of afraid of heights. I'm not thrilled with bridges, either, but if I need to be on the other side of the bridge, then I'll go over the bridge. Now my fear is other-centered. All of my fears are external. I fear for my son Richard's life [her remaining child]. I never fear for my own, which drives him a little bit nuts. Maybe it's because, while I'm afraid of any pain associated with death, I can't wait to see Colleen and Steve again. So, I'm good either way."

CALL FOR BACKUP IF YOU NEED IT

It is not a sign of failure if this is something you can't do on your own. Many people who have struggled with fear-based issues and anxiety need outside professional help to work on themselves. Therapy is something I pooh-poohed in my immature past, but I have seen so many people benefit from the myriad treatments out there, like exposure therapy (no, you don't get naked; get your mind out of the gutter—in this practice, you are gradually exposed to your fear) and group therapy. Choose what works best for you—and realize you have already made the hardest choice: deciding to face your fears rather than avoid them.

Bottom line: If there is anything I want you to take away from this chapter, it's this: Courage is action in the face of fear. Or as Winston Churchill put it: "Fear is a reaction. Courage is a decision." One you get over fear, you can forge your new normal.

A New Normal

Your Vulnerability Is Your Strength

I left out one big fear factor in the previous chapter on purpose. It is such a looming issue that I needed to devote an entire chapter to it. That's the fear of vulnerability. "Vulnerability" is defined as the ability or the chance of being physically or emotionally wounded. In the military, we don't like vulnerability, since it can imply that you're in danger or in a weak position. Being vulnerable was the very thing you didn't want to be as a soldier, after all. When a soldier is in a vulnerable position, you can get killed. Vulnerable to the enemy. Vulnerable to attack. We were trained not to be vulnerable. Yet, in "real life," it takes on a slightly different meaning. While being vulnerable on the battlefield means weakness, being vulnerable with yourself doesn't have to mean you're weak. It can, in fact, mean the opposite. Being vulnerable is strength. It means to be fully open to others, expressing true feelings, or, as in our PATHH program, what we call being authentic. It is not about oversharing or being overly emotional; it is about showing who you are under all that armor. Everybody has feelings, as much as they try to hide them, and while it is scary to be vulnerable, courage is acknowledging vulnerability. Vulnerability has gotten the short end of the stick for too long.

It was understandable, therefore, that I hadn't had a good handle on my own vulnerability, given all my years in the army. So when it came to that moment of me staring at that photo of the younger me in my in-laws' bedroom, it was hard to identify what I was feeling. I did know I needed to come to grips with that new person in the mirror. I thought I had done all the healing in the hospital. Little did I know that the real work was only beginning. I had to look at that old image of Travis and let go of that version of him. Otherwise, clinging to that old life, clinging to old patterns and old beliefs that were stymieing my future, fearful of moving on, was going to stymie that caterpillar from morphing into a butterfly.

When I was still Staff Sargent Mills at the hospital, still an active member of the army, I couldn't wait to retire. My goal was to get out of the hospital and go on with life and just live. However, when that day finally came, I had no idea who I was going to *be*. I was lost. I didn't know how to interact with Chloe as a father or Kelsey as a husband. I didn't know how to interact with people outside the safety bubble of Walter Reed. I would go to the grocery store, and little kids would come up to me wide-eyed and curious, and ask their mother, "What happened to his legs, Mom?" not aware that I could hear them. At first, I had no idea how to react to it. I didn't know how to deal with people staring at me.

It was fate that I met David Vobora at that birthday party in Dallas in early 2014. David, who owned a gym in town, was working with the NFL and Olympic athletes at the time, and we found ourselves sipping some whiskey together in the host's kitchen.

"When was the last time you worked out?" David asked me.

"Hey, I don't want to make you feel like an idiot, but I don't have arms and legs," I responded, to get a laugh.

"I don't care if you don't have arms and legs—you're a living, breathing human and we can tap into your physicality. Why don't we redefine that? What are you afraid of?"

And that, my friends, is what started my real journey back into physical health. David opened up his personal gym to me, offering his training expertise. While he hadn't trained an amputee before, he did his research and customized and adapted workouts to the unique challenges posed by my injuries. We tried different exercises—some worked, some failed miserably, terribly—but we tried them. We found a rhythm that suited me, and I could feel myself getting stronger. Beyond the physical improvements, I could see that I was becoming more comfortable with my new abbreviated body, as well as becoming more comfortable in my own skin out in the real world, because the Walter Reed world was a bubble of safety.

He helped me work out in ways I never knew I could. It was amazing to see how my physical change helped me transform mentally as well. David saw it too. "With all those sessions, I could see that Travis went to those vulnerable places. He was becoming more comfortable with who he was."

Indeed, I was getting a handle on how this body of mine could find its way. But the sessions also gave me something else: a sense of getting back into a routine that gave me a sense of normalcy I hadn't felt in a long time. I would go to David's for a workout, then I go to over to my friend Reese's house (he was my business manager at the time), and we would talk about work and booking speaking engagements. I looked forward to this daily routine I didn't even know I was craving a month earlier. I was carving out a new normal.

This is exactly what I needed at the time. I needed to know that I could still do things that have self-worth and that life outside of the normal life was going to be okay. It made me see that no matter what you face and go through, you can get back to a sense of normalcy. And that sense of normalcy is something we all crave: I kept on wondering, *How can I fit back into society?* I craved that feeling of the everyday. This is when I learned that what I was craving was really about my mind wanting to be in a state of balance. This is also called homeostasis, the maintaining of internal balance and equilibrium in the body and its various functions. Just as our body likes equilibrium, our mind likes it too. And then the more confident I got, the more comfortable I became in my own skin (even though there was less of it). A great example of this was during the pandemic, when studies indicated that we can recover even if still in a state of stress. They also showed that humans can establish a new normal even while still being stressed, whereas previous studies indicated that recovery would only start only after the stress is removed.[1] This goes to show that we can be resilient even when we are still going through some headwinds.

And this working out and building my confidence helped me with my interactions with other people. Kelsey saw how my mood shifted, my friends could tell that I was managing better, and I even handled strangers better too. Once, soon after working with David, a nine-year-old child asked me, "Where'd your arm go?" which was followed up by his embarrassed mom apologizing for her son's imposition. "I am so sorry! He doesn't know what he is saying!"

"Oh, no, don't worry about it," I told her; and to her son, I showed him a newly discovered magic trick: spinning my new motorized hand. I finally was at a place where I understood people will always look. If I were them, I would too. Now having come to grips my "new normal," I figured I might as well own it.

In fact, I am even better than normal—to a group of kids, I am like Ironman with my bionic arms and legs. And my daughter and son don't remember me any other way—so my body is completely natural to them.

IT TAKES PRACTICE

It has been years since my injury, yet I still have a hard time with the whole vulnerability thing. But that is okay—it's not like you wake up one day and proclaim, "Look at that—I am an expert at being vulnerable!" It takes regular practice. I still have work to do, as I often find myself going back to old habits and hiding my feelings, especially around strangers. For example, I still deflect my feelings by using humor, making a joke. It is a very effective mask, and I try to be aware of it when I am doing it. Some board up their feelings with perfectionism or cynicism—my go-to is humor.

Once you are vulnerable, only then can you have *agency*, just like Pam had in "Principle #8." That's the power in feeling in control over our actions. Having a sense of normalcy brings with it a sense of being in control over what is happening, which all adds to our having agency over our lives. Kristen Neff puts it this way: "The safer people feel, the more open and flexible they can be in response to their environment."[2] This feeling of getting power back is really what agency is all about. Basically, you are back in the driver's seat, and you can take control over your life. That is what I want for you.

Here are three ways to help you get agency:

1. Make a commitment to make a positive change in your life—and not someone else's version of what that looks like. Not your mom's, your dad's, your wife's, not even your dog's version of what that should look like.
2. Create an action plan. When I had things to do every day, it gave me a routine, which then gave me a sense of normalcy so I could finally think about my future. The routine also let me feel that things were "normal."
3. Reflect on how that plan is going. If it is not going as well as you hoped, look at another way to change course.

I believe that once you have agency, you can be truly vulnerable. Maybe you never needed to be vulnerable before. But after a loss or a setback, you will need it to be able to move forward. You can't pass GO if you don't. It may take time, and you'll need to come from a place that feels safe. In our PATHH program, we tell our participants that they are in a place that is safe. They can say whatever they want to say, and it won't leave the room. (It's out version of "What happens in Vegas stays in Vegas.") So, every guest can feel completely open to be vulnerable with one another. It's not easy. In between the hard discussions, we do some lighter activities, such as archery, meditation, or some creative arts. They will spend some hard minutes trying to regulate their emotions, because a lot of these stories are going to access things that they haven't accessed, sometimes in years. We get them to a place where they can see past the struggle and forge their own new normal.

ROI Decision-Making

I found a great tool in helping me get perspective on a problem. I ask myself, *Is this important? Is it solvable?* If not, what is plan B? What is the ROI (return on investment) on one plan of action versus another? Having detachment from the issue will help you get perspective—sometimes removing yourself from the situation or giving yourself some time will help you figure out what is important. "The solution to a problem is not going to be found *in* the problem. You have to get outside of it to make an assessment and find a solution," my pal Jocko Willink has smartly said to me, more than once.

BEING VULNERABLE IS GOOD FOR YOU

Science shows that if our emotional system is taxed, so is our nervous system. And since everything is connected, we can see that toll manifest in ailments like panic attacks, chronic pain, gastrointestinal issues, immune disorders, and chronic anxiety and depression.[3] There is a feedback loop between our brain and our body; what happens to us, how we process it in our brain, can affect how our body reacts. I have also seen the effects of PTSD a hundred times over, although the military doesn't have a monopoly on it. Any which way, fear will only proceed to take over your life if you don't stop it in tracks.

I connected to David Vobora so much because he had his own battles and came out better for it: He was playing for the Seattle Seahawks when a series of shoulder injuries in 2011 ended his career. David had struggled with an identity crisis of no longer being on the football field, as well as the fear that came with not knowing what the future held. He was at the top of his game, and suddenly, bang, he was ripped from that. His whole world turned upside down, with very little to help him transition well. Having been prescribed opioids for his physical pain but nothing to help him cope mentally, he began a slow downhill slide into addiction. He spiraled, spending thousands of dollars a week avoiding withdrawal, until the day his girlfriend (now wife) found him hanging off the edge of a twentieth-floor hotel balcony, threatening to jump. This was the proverbial wake-up call (although he doesn't remember any of it), and he finally sought help.

"I went through a seven-day detox, where I crapped myself, lost 34 pounds, and had two seizures. At one point, I tried to lift a plate of food but instead dropped it, where it shattered all over the floor. I was trying to pick up the shards out of embarrassment when the nurses rushed in—they thought I may try to use the broken pieces to cut myself. Before I knew it, I was tied to a bed, wondering, *What the hell? How did I get here?*

"That week was brutal, but I got to the other side. And it took several years and a lot of work and forgiveness to keep on the other side, but eventually, I came to the realization that my addiction was based on fear. I was sexually abused when I was ten, which I stuffed so deep down I couldn't even recall it. But today, I see that I used football and the adoration of others to escape from facing this trauma. I had put up a facade to mask the fear."

Like David, Ray also struggled with his identity when he retired. When he left the service, he had a hard landing back into civilian life, struggled with anxiety, and tended to self-isolate, staying home with his wife and avoiding social situations that would make him feel uncomfortable. He wasn't dealing with a host of emotions that were boiling within him—he struggled a lot with a lost sense of identity and PTSD. (Ray is not alone in his struggles with emotion—many who have PTSD are scared to show emotion because it means a loss of control.) For Ray, these repressed emotions revealed themselves in a full-blown panic attack.

"One day at home, I was at the landing of the second floor of my house, about to walk down the stairs, and all of a sudden, I couldn't feel my legs. My lungs closed up as I gasped for air. I stood there like a statue, afraid to move. Finally, I managed to call out for my wife, who raced up the stairs and helped me crawl down. As we sat at the bottom of the stairs, I tried to catch my breath. She sat next to me, rubbing my back, and I eventually calmed down. I saw a doctor later that week and found out that I had had a panic attack. I had experienced a physical manifestation of everything I was feeling inside."

Ray is a living, breathing example of just how much the body is connected to the mind and how holding in our emotions can affect us. He hid his vulnerability. Although it wasn't an easy road, and it wasn't until he attended the Warrior PATHH Program and learned wellness and regulation practices that his panic attacks gradually subsided.

Like David, Ray, and me, anyone going through a tough time may not want to show any fear or sadness, but holding on to them, letting them eat away at you, or shoving them into the back corners of your mind can be way more dangerous than showing them. Thank God they both got help and are in much better places for it—and now are helping others do the same.

GETTING USED TO YOUR NEW NORMAL

To be truly vulnerable, Brené Brown says, is to be afraid and courageous at same time. What does she mean by that? New things are going to take courage, and it is okay to feel scared. Someone once said to me to consider that feeling scared is really about feeling excited. It is your body saying that something is happening, and it's preparing you to do something extraordinary. Isn't that a cool way to look at it? Transitioning out to the military was that signal for me that I was going on to do something extraordinary. But I needed the old Travis to die, metaphorically speaking, so that the new Travis could move onto a path that would be so much greater. Don't get to a point in your life where you start thinking, "I shoulda, woulda, coulda." When thinking about a new normal—what do you want that to look like? My new normal includes my wife and kids. It includes my businesses. It includes all the work I do for my foundation. What will drive your new normal? Whatever you do, don't let the fear of the future—of the unknown, of a new normal—get in the way of vulnerability. Because that armor is keeping away everything you want in life.

PRINCIPLE #11

Serve

Find Your Voice, Build on Your Strengths, and Live Meaningfully

As I lay in that hospital bed those first few weeks after the injury, I often asked myself why I was spared. Fast-forward through nineteen months of rehab at Walter Reed, where the amazing staff helped this twenty-five-year-old baby walk, dress, and eat again, I realized I was given another chance to see the opportunities in front of me. At first, I was *that guy* with no arms or legs—there were only two of us at the hospital at that time. (There were five total throughout the Afghanistan/Iraq war; I was fourth.) I stood out, and for that reason,

I realize now how my extraordinary injury gave me a certain power. Because I was so recognizable, anywhere I went on the hospital campus—to the gym, to the cafeteria, or in hospital hallways—I was the physical embodiment of a miraculous survival story. And that power gave me a purpose: I realized I could, by example, help injured soldiers understand that life goes on no matter what. And that felt good. I was a man on a mission: Anyone there would attest to my unbowed determination to get out of there as soon as I could, but I was also motivated by motivating others. Much like the Kesha dance parties I instigated, I felt an instinctual need to provide a lighter side of things when things felt dark. When I wasn't in the rehab center, I started visiting soldiers like me, who had come into Walter Reed's doors (nearly) as messed up as I was. I'd meet them in their rooms, and tell them, "Hi, I am Travis, and I want you to know you are going to be fine." I did the same thing that Todd Nicely did for me all those months earlier. I knew what it meant to be seen, and more important, to see someone just like me. I did this enough and got a little reputation for being the welcome committee, acquiring the nickname "the Mayor of 62" (after the rehab building we lived in).

Therapists would ask me to come by the MATC (Military Advanced Training Center) to help someone who needed a pep talk. One particular day, there was a double amputee who was so afraid of falling that he wouldn't walk off a 4-inch step, even with the help of a Solo-Step harness.

"It's okay, bud; how long you've been here for?" I asked him after a little introduction from a physical therapist.

"Since December." Wow, he had been here six months before me. I could tell Kerry was frustrated that he wasn't trying.

"You know what we're gonna do?" I said. "We're gonna go down that four-inch step today. You are amazing. I know you can do it."

"No, I can't do it." He halted.

I pushed him off the step. Don't worry—he was okay, as he was safely secured in the harness. I wanted to show him that he was safe.

"Look, you are okay right?"

He nodded. I could see relief in his eyes.

"Now you do it without me pushing you. Lean on me, buddy, lean on my shoulder."

He did, and after a few missteps, he conquered that step. Success!

"Do you realize you are literally leaning on a quadruple amputee?!" Kerry exclaimed, noting the irony of the moment.

That guy—and many like him—was experiencing what I had experienced, but he had a bit more difficulty in seeing past his injury. I was glad to be of help. It gave me a sense of purpose, which I needed at that time. I now realize I was experiencing the most important piece of post-traumatic growth: Once you stop looking inward, you can start working outward.

When you have taken care of yourself, you can help others. Here you are, the final step of healing—finding purpose. It took me a while after my injury to see my purpose before me, but heck, if I hadn't, I may not have started the foundation, and I may not have helped hundreds of other amputees. I lost my sense of purpose on the battlefield, but I found it again, in a different place.

Listen, you get one go-round in life, one chance to make an impact. Maybe that impact is being a coach and giving your all to the students or being a counselor who can help other people like yourself get through something tough. There is a wonderful corner you'll turn, from feeling helpless to helping others. Take my PATHH guides Ray and James, who each had to rebuild their identity when they retired from service; both found it in helping others overcome their trauma experiences. Or Dave Vobora, who pivoted his upside-down career-ending injury into a lifelong vocation of helping those who have physical challenges get in their best shape of their lives. What are you good at? What can you do to help others in need? How can you make your own little corner of the world better? This is the beauty of post-traumatic growth. It can be as simple as being there for a friend.

Or a stranger. James, who credited two marine pals for pulling him out of his hole and getting him involved in a veterans motorcycle club, remembers the night he saved someone.

He had been at a party at a local bar with a few other guys from the club, and he was leaving when he heard a weird noise coming from around the corner of the building.

"So, I walked around, and there was this guy, curled up in the fetal position on the concrete, just bawling. He was one of the marines who had been in the bar earlier and was on the struggle bus. I stayed out there with him. We sat on the street curb and just talked for two hours. When I first walked up to him, he wanted to kill himself. By the time we departed, he didn't. That made me feel really good—probably the best I had felt since before I even joined the Marine Corps. And it was an addictive feeling. It was a tinge of happiness—something that I hadn't found in a long time."

That night, James realized that once he started stepping out of his own trauma, he found that he could help others who were waging battles in the head like he did. James found that he craved to have that feeling of goodness again, so he would seek out situations where he felt that he could be of use, which is ironic as he has been known to say that talking with people is his least favorite thing in the world to do (which I find hard to believe). He eventually went on to get his degree in recreational therapy, which helps patients with physical and emotional trauma through creative activities and helps them develop skills for daily living. "I knew right away I didn't want to work in a hospital—I wanted to work with vets. Long story, but I did both of my internships at the Travis Mills Foundation, and here I am several years later."

PTG IN ACTION

I am no expert, so I point to PATHH founder Josh Goldberg, who wrote *Struggle Well*, the seminal book on PTG,[1] to better explain how this happens: "A great deal of the time people who go through these difficult life experiences—these traumas and these losses—often reported in the aftermath of that experience going through the process of posttraumatic growth. This leads them to report that their life had changed for the better in terms of it being more authentic and more meaningful and more purposeful than it was before they had that experience. They talk about growing in terms of their sense of hope for their future, a recognition of the value of deeper relationships with other people, a sense of personal strength—the idea that nothing can permanently knock us down; an appreciation for the small and big things in life; and spiritual and existential growth—the idea that they are now asking and reflecting upon the deepest questions that life can offer us: who am I, why am I here, and where do I belong? And that's what posttraumatic growth describes, and what the entire science and concept behind it are all about."

It's as if a metamorphosis takes place and you rebuild yourself from the inside out. And once that happens, you can start to look outward to help others, whether that is immediate family or friends or a larger community. But by starting small, you'll see where your passion lies. You will see that this growth will give you the means to find fulfillment with helping others. Find meaning out of other ashes of your trauma. This is one of the beautiful things about post-traumatic growth—that one can see growth after struggle. One of the founders of the PTG movement, Richard Tedeschi, PhD, has said that "people develop a new understanding of themselves, the world they live in, how to relate to other people, the kind of future they might have and a better understanding of how to live life."[2]

With this kind of growth, you'll get to see what is important in life and what isn't. It isn't easy, forging this new path. Believe me, there have been struggles and doubts along the way, especially when I first started my foundation. There have been sleepless nights when I tossed and turned, asking myself, *Who the heck do I think I am, starting a foundation from scratch?* But by morning, I'd wake up and think to myself, *Why not me? I may not be here tomorrow, so why don't I do everything I can?* It has been ten great years without my legs, so why stop now?

The idea of giving back, of helping out those in need, started out small. We began sending out care packages. And then we thought, *Let's do something bigger and better.* And we moved to Maine, and thanks to many donors, we transformed the former Elizabeth Arden estate into a paradise where families of recalibrated soldiers can come and enjoy time together and with other veterans. Here is the best payoff to resilience:

giving back and offering a sanctuary for others to build their own. I found purpose by helping vets like me at Walter Reed and later through TMF, but no one needs to start a foundation to pass on the strength they built to do something good in their lives.

FIND YOUR VOICE

On the one hand, trauma victims have struggled to feel that they have a voice; on the other, they rightly perceive that their voice will not be heard, or at least not respected. With post-traumatic growth, many people regain their voice—or, for those like Pam Swan, find it for the first time. When Pam, whom we met in the "Principle #8" chapter, had been brought back home after she and her brother attempted to run away, she did settle back into school, where she had always felt safe. She was a sophomore taking a home economics class when she heard they were going to cut the class and let go of its teacher because the district didn't have enough funding for it. She couldn't believe it. There was going to be a board meeting that night, so she went.

"I settled into the third row of the auditorium and listened to all the excuses as to why they were going to get rid of this class and the teacher who taught it. I really liked this teacher—she had taught me things that I never learned at home (but should have): sewing, cooking, even balancing a checkbook (although

I am not sure my parents even had one). So, I really wanted to be there for her. When the board opened up the meeting for comment, I stood up. There were several classmates sitting in nearby rows; I felt their eyes on me. My legs started shaking, and I thought, *I'm not gonna get the words out.* I don't remember exactly what I said, but the gist was, 'I wish you would think of the economics of where we live, this small town—and how many people in this high school will end up staying here needing to know the basics of how to cook, how to balance checkbooks, how to take care of a home…and you're taking that away from them and putting dollars in a music program. Of course, music is important, but the odds of somebody from this town ending up playing for some orchestra in a big city is pretty small; that person would be much better served knowing how to care for their family and home closer to home.'

"I am not sure how I got through all that without my knees buckling, but the next thing I remember, the board members were getting out of their chairs to give me standing ovation. Members of the audience got up too. They decided to keep the class, and the teacher. I couldn't believe I changed something for the better. I went home feeling so proud that I had done a good thing."

Looking back on it now, Pam sees that although she was still young, she had found her voice. It wasn't too much later after this that she moved out of her parents' home and got a job—all made possible because of that home ec course. She had proven to herself that she could live better and financially more stable because of that class, and she almost certainly helped many people in her community by saving that class.

BECOME MORE EMPATHETIC

Having empathy for others is a common theme in PTG. Take Kim, an LA-native mother of one, who had been long married to an absent husband. Several years ago, she went through two bouts of non-Hodgkin's lymphoma. As she soldiered on, taking care of her daughter when her husband was often away on business, she faced her cancer mostly alone. Sometimes, it just got to be too much, and she found a source of comfort in drinking. She eventually divorced, becoming a single mom responsible for raising and providing for her daughter. A glass of wine a night turned into two, then into a bottle. It went on for years. "Even within a couple of years after the second cancer, I was passing out on the couch every night after drinking a bottle to a bottle and a half of wine. There was one night when I woke up, dark and quiet in my bedroom, knowing that beyond my door was my lovely daughter sleeping in her own room. I thought, *What does my daughter think of me? What am I doing to her by not even being present for her? I must be screwing her up for life.* I was at the breaking point. I woke up the next day and cried, knowing I just couldn't do this anymore. It's ironic in a way, since I tried everything in my power to stay alive during both battles with cancer. I did everything I could to fight that, but thought, *Here you are, killing yourself with alcohol.*"

She got herself into AA and continues to go, after years of sobriety. Even for people who don't go through a physical trauma like her, healing through an emotional trauma can make you feel like a new person after you've done all the work, especially something like AA. It was as if she was shedding her old skin. When this sort of transformation happens, you gain perspective and empathy that you now can carry over to others. And Kim did just that. She had a friend, Mary, who was having a hard time with the loss of her son. He had died in a car accident two years prior, but she was having difficulty with it, so much so that she often thought about suicide. Everyone deals with grief differently, and while some people would have told Mary that she needed to move on, Kim didn't. She was there for her and allowed her to be as vulnerable as she wanted to be. For Kim, sobriety will always be a journey—she is still learning every day—but the realization that she has done the work on herself so she can be of help to other people keeps her going.

On both a macro and a micro level, people can turn their struggles into something positive that pays it forward to those who may just be getting started on their road to recovery. I'm a believer that everything happens for a reason. Those who are injured and suffering have every right to just take care of themselves until they heal; others sometimes make a choice to

care for others over their own needs while they are still healing. Either way, embracing post-traumatic growth will give you
a new perspective on our goals and aspirations we may have
lost sight of in the fog of trauma. But once that lifts, there is
an opportunity to be who you really are. So, go out there, be
authentic, figure out who you want to be, and don't be afraid of
what other people think of you. Serve something greater than
yourself.

Like I said, at the end of the day, you get one go-round in
life. You get one chance to make your mark. How do you want
to leave your mark on this world? This answer should give you
purpose. If that's being a coach and giving your all to the students, or being a parent, and being the best darn parent there
is, then how can you be better at that every day?

Now, let's figure out a plan for that and execute it.

Make It a Daily Practice

Ask Yourself: What Is Stopping Me from Recalibrating?

Resilience isn't something that you get, like a sticker or a badge, and then you carry it around for life. You need to continue to work at it, and you will want to, because we will all need it—again and again. Hopefully by now you have learned that pain is good and important—never fun or easy, but we can learn from it. And build a resilience for it. Science shows that we can develop and improve our resilience—but it requires practice and consistency. What we discuss in this final chapter will help build on what you have learned in this book.

These are built within three pillars of practice: choice, control, and compassion.

EVERY DAY IS A CHOICE

Humans make about thirty-five thousand conscious decisions each day.[1] Each decision, of course, can change your life, in big ways and small, for better or worse. While I couldn't stop that IED from doing its job that day, I can stop it from detracting from the rest of my life. From those decisions, you have a choice of how to react. Do you choose to be angry, isolated, fearful, untrusting? Or do you choose to be hopeful, fearless, and trusting? You need the mental capacity, that space, to make good decisions. So, the key to being resilient is giving yourself space. Give yourself some self-compassion; realize, yes, life sucks sometimes. Here are some things that I do to give myself that mental space so that I can better handle making choices with any of life's curveballs...or cyclones.

Ask yourself five questions. After a loss, shakeup, or trauma, you will have a lot of questions. Much as we talk about in the "Principle #2" chapter, you don't want to get stuck on "why," but rather think about how you want to live your life moving forward. Questions should help you reflect, not ruminate. Liz, when she was faced with the death of her husband, had a choice to make, and she asked herself what kind of parent she would be to her kids. She made the decision that her kids wouldn't lose both of their parents that day. She made this decision very quickly, as a young widow at thirty-three, based on reflection and asking herself hard questions. What follows are five go-to questions I always ask myself when going through something tough.

1. What happened? Focus on the who, what, where, when, and why. But not too much on the why.
2. How do I feel that this happened? It is okay to be angry. Acknowledge your feelings.
3. What understanding can be gleaned from what happened? Did I react badly or did I react appropriately?
4. How can I learn from it?
5. What is my plan to move forward?

Remember, goals work. Studies show that people who set goals are more likely to achieve those goals.[2] Why? Well, it has something to do with the brain's neuroplasticity, which means that our noodle can rewire itself depending on outside stimuli, such as learning a new language. Setting goals is another way you can make your brain adapt, thereby helping you focus on what you really want to get done and giving you direction and the motivation for you to achieve it.

Commit to your goals. Reality check: The percentage of people who set goals and follow through with them is pretty low—so, the beauty is in the follow-through. A 2015 study showed that when people wrote down their goals, they were 33 percent more successful in achieving them than were those who formulated outcomes in their head.[3] Every once in a while—every day, every week, whatever works for you—check in with yourself and see if you are sticking to your goals or if you need to readjust.

EVERY DAY IS ABOUT CONTROL

We read earlier how much resilience is about controlling our emotions. But that can be easier said than done, I know. One of the core feelings that people have is an unshakable loss of control. A major plot point in this book is that you can't change what happened, nor make it go away, but you can control your attitude. After all, you don't want to fall into the category of learned helplessness or victimhood. Here are a few ways to stave off helplessness:

Be optimistic. Are you a glass half-full or glass half-empty type of person? If you are a glass half-empty, time to change up things. Negativity is only going to hurt your chances of building resilience. Negative feelings, as well as feelings of anger and fear, will not help you get out of your situation; they will actually only keep you stuck in the situation longer. So again, make the choice to be more optimistic. Studies show that optimism and resilience go hand in hand, as optimistic people display more resilience when facing difficult situations.[4] Not naturally someone who always sees the bright side of things? Here are a few ways to practice being more positive:

- While you may not be someone who believes "everything happens for a reason," is there something you can learn from the experience? Knowing that you come away from a bad experience with more knowledge and wisdom is a powerful thing.

- When a negative thought comes into your head, try to turn it into something positive. Instead of "I can't believe this happened to me," say instead, "Okay, this happened to me, but I am still alive. I am still breathing and living."

- Everyone who knows me knows that I am a joker. Humor lightens the mood and can make a tense situation immediately better. But there is a right way and a wrong way to be funny. Goodhearted and witty humor is good for you and others; "maladaptive" humor—using put-downs and derisive comments—and aggressive sarcasm can be unhealthy.[5] Watch what you say and how you say it.

Have a creative outlet. Whether it is music, painting, writing, belly dancing, or model ship building, having an outlet to help you get out of your head is one of the best things you can do to manage emotions. James is a big believer in drawing.

While he was going through recovery, all his creations were super dark, and only in black-and-white. Think skulls and devils and destruction. "Because I was looking at life through the lens of my path. And it wasn't until after PATHH that art became something fun for me. I do it with my family now, like draw pictures of fish and trees...." Art helped him process so much that he could not process through words. Journaling is another great way to process your emotions, as well as track progress and practice gratitude. Being creative is being curious.

Get walking. Any exercise is shown to help with our moods and overall health. If you do it outside, even better. When Bobby gets too inside his head, he likes to take what he calls "mindless" walks outside—on a trail, by the river, wherever to clear his head. He has the right idea to get outside. Spending time outside in the fresh air and also surrounded by trees and nature—a practice the Japanese call "forest bathing" or *shinrin yoku*—is in fact becoming a hot trend in wellness circles. Why? It has been shown to lower blood pressure, decrease anxiety and depression, and increase overall well-being and creativity.[6] There is also a 2019 study in *Scientific Reports* that found spending at least two hours in nature every week resulted in better overall well-being and health.[7] (So basically, your mom, who would always tell you to go outside and play, was on to something.)

While you're at it, walk to the gym. Why not get your mental health in shape while you're getting your body in shape?

There have long been studies that show how exercise can be good for your mental health in general, but there is growing evidence that it can particularly help those in trauma recovery and those with PTSD.[8] Regular exercise can help alleviate symptoms of anxiety, depression, sleep issues, and other PTSD symptoms.[9] Whether it's the physicality of punching a bag, lifting heavy weights, or focusing on balancing one leg in a yoga pose that does it, that experience of endurance and strength can make you feel tougher and more flexible in life outside the gym.

Be grateful. We have a whole chapter on gratitude, but it is worth repeating here since it can be so important to our resilience. It should really be practiced every day. A University of Pennsylvania study found when people considered their positive experiences, they were more likely to be inspired to take future altruistic action—contributing toward others' happiness.[10] The US Army recently incorporated practices of gratitude in its Comprehensive Soldier Fitness program, developed with Martin Seligman and the University of Pennsylvania's Positive Psychology Center.[11] Research shows "hunting the good stuff," trying to find things every day to be thankful for, can counteract negative emotions, while benefiting your health and sleep and improving relationships.[12] This exercise can also help us pay attention to how we are feeling emotionally, so when things start to feel a little bit off of control, we can reel it back in rather than falling into a state of fear or anxiety.

Challenge yourself to think of one thing that you're grateful for every day, but make it matter—if it's your kids, don't just write "my kids." For me, I may say, one day, "I am so glad that my son, Dax, got to play in the pool with me today." Challenge yourself to think about what specifically you're particularly grateful for—that your kids are developing into respectful people? Gratitude makes us appreciate what we have, instead of focusing on what we don't have. It improves our physical health and well-being, in addition to our mental health.

CONNECT, EVERY DAY

Connection is so important to maintaining our resilience. Our support groups—our friends, family, dog, whoever—are our buffer zones to life's catastrophes. It's the friend you can call any time of day and they will pick up. It's the parent who will tell you the things you need to hear when you have a bad day. It's the girlfriend who makes you a mean chicken noodle soup when you have a bad cold. It's the dog who stares at you because it just loves you unconditionally. So, make sure those lines of communication remain open at all times. For me, I love being an entrepreneur who gives back: besides my foundation, I am always looking for a good business to invest in my community. I have a lodge, a restaurant, and a taproom—I love being part of the community in which I live.

Up Your EI

One of the best ways of staying connected is having a high emotional intelligence (EI), sort of another word for being empathetic. It's the ability to understand and control our emotions and sympathize with the emotions of others. It makes us empathic to those around us, which in turn will improve our relationships. It's a two-way street: We strengthen our own self-esteem by expressing affection and comradery in our relationships, which further strengthens our connections. By feeling connected, we feel stronger and are better able to rebound from trauma. Here are some go-tos for getting yourself more connected and gaining some EI.

Be social. I am not talking about Facebook or TikTok here. Those will only usurp your resilience, if you ask me. I am talking about your IRL relationships. (My kids taught me that.) Parents, siblings, high school friends, work colleagues, neighbors, children. Who are the ones you can count on during a crisis? Who is your do-or-die team? Can you list two? Ten? Quantity doesn't matter, quality does. If you think you are lacking in this department, can you ask yourself why you think that is? Have you been isolating yourself? Are you fearful of relationships because of past trauma? If you feel ready to open your circle, think of places where you could meet some like-minded people. Athletic groups or intramural sports, book clubs, volunteering—you will soon see that we are surrounded by good people.

Ask hard questions. If you are feeling isolated or disconnected from people, it is a good time to check in with yourself: How are you with yourself and with others? Are you particularly hard on yourself or get upset when things don't go your way? Do you expect too much from others and get mad if they don't live up to expectations? Or do you bury everything inside? Do you hide your feelings and let them fester? If you said yes to any of these, what do you think you should do about it?

Understand the difference between being alone and being isolated. Sometimes, people feel like if they are around people all the time, they won't feel the hurt. They avoid their feelings because they are never alone with them. But they will only fester that way. Being alone is a great time to think and problem-solve. No matter what you are going through in your own tough journey, I know the worst part can be when everybody's gone. It's just you. And I still struggle with this to this day, sometimes at night when questions like to creep in and my mind starts racing. But this is when resilience will really come in handy. Ask the hard questions to yourself and be honest. Having a good social circle is great for resilience, but so is alone time.

Find your spirit. I'm not your typical Sunday-morning, church-going guy. I have my own way of talking to the man upstairs, and I was very angry with him at one point. Okay. Very, very angry. Lying in bed in Walter Reed, my sister-in-law had brought me a plaque that read: DO NOT BE AFRAID FOR

GOD WALKS BESIDE YOU. She hung it on the wall next to my bed, and since I couldn't move too much at this point, I was forced to read it over and over. One morning, when I couldn't take it anymore, I told my mom, "Hey, can you take that off the wall or turn it over? I'm tired of reading it. I mean, where was God that day when I got blown up?"

My mom replied, "Travis, quit that talk." And she refused to turn it over or remove it. I couldn't get up and do it myself. But maybe it was a good thing, after all, that I had to look at it: I had to try to understand the whole madness of what happened. And I realized I was blessed to have lived through an injury that most die from. That is when hope started to set in: I began to understand that I was given the ability to still *live*. No matter your religion, whom you pray to, or what you believe in, have hope in what is to come, not what has happened, and have faith in yourself, as well as having faith in others.

So much about gaining and maintaining resilience is about practicing it. And life gives us many opportunities to do so, am I right? If you try to be resilient every day, it will become second nature, and with that inevitable next crisis or challenge, you will be that much stronger and prepared to take it on. It will be about how to put one foot in front of the other to keep you going. Always bounce back.

EPILOGUE: A RECALIBRATED LIFE

I don't remember who first told me about this metaphor, but it has stuck with me ever since. There is a traditional Japanese craft called *kintsugi* (from the Japanese words *kin* and *tsugi*, meaning "golden joinery"), which is the art of carefully repairing broken pottery with lacquer mixed with gold or silver. The result is a piece that is more beautiful and embellished than it had been before.

That is how I feel about being recalibrated. I was pasted back together, with metal parts glued back on, but I became a better person because of my being broken and doing all that repair work. That is post-traumatic growth.

I may have scars—like those beautiful lines of lacquer on a vase—but I am healed. I am healed as much as I am going to heal. I am not going to grow my arms and legs back (although that would be pretty cool, wouldn't it?), but I found my "new normal." I never feel sorry for what I went through because I wouldn't be the person I am today if I hadn't gone through what I did.

As you finish this book, I want you to leave with this message: You are a lot more resilient than you think you are. And there are things that you can choose to do to allow that resilience to bloom. Are you ready to make that choice?

ACKNOWLEDGMENTS

would be nothing—NOTHING—without my wife, Kelsey, and my two amazing children, Chloe and Dax. They are my world. I'd like to thank them for making me a better person. I completely believe that my recovery, as well as my success in life, is because of them being on my side, cheering me forward!!

I would also like to thank my parents, Dennis and Cheri Mills, as well as Craig and Tammy Buck. They have also showed up in so many ways—I am forever grateful.

For all those who helped make this book what it is with their stories, I am forever indebted: Tuesday's Children, Lorree Sutton, Cristyne Nichols and her team; Toddy Nicely, David Vobora, Kerri Quinn, Emma, Laura, Kim, Liz, Mitch, Robert, Jenn, and Mike. A special shout out to my TMF staff, especially James Prindle, who added so much heart to this book, and also to Ray Edgar and Kelly Rosenberry. Thank you for being so candid. Thank you to Josh Goldberg Ken Falke for creating the amazing PATHH program that helps so many people.

To Rick Richter, my agent, who always believes in me and my message, to Kathryn Huck, who helped me shape that message into an amazing book, and to Dan Ambrosino and all the people at Hachette who helped me get my book into the hands of people who need it.

NOTES

INTRODUCTION

1.   www.thenationalcouncil.org, accessed March 23, 2023, https://www
.thenationalcouncil.org/wp-content/uploads/2022/08/Trauma-infographic
.pdf.

2.   Alyssa Fowers and William Wan, "A Third of Americans Now
Show Signs of Clinical Anxiety or Depression, Census Bureau Finds amid
Coronavirus Pandemic," *Washington Post*, May 26, 2020.

PRINCIPLE #1

1.   Bryan E. Robinson, "Why You Hate Uncertainty, and How to Cope,"
Psychology Today, November 6, 2020, https://www.psychologytoday.com/gb
/blog/the-right-mindset/202011/why-you-hate-uncertainty-and-how-cope.

2.   Tanja Michael et al., "Rumination in Posttraumatic Stress Disorder,"
Depression and Anxiety 24, no. 5 (October 13, 2006): 307–317, https://pubmed
.ncbi.nlm.nih.gov/17041914/.

3.   Martin E. P. Seligman, Andrew R. Allen, and Paul B. Lester,
"PTSD: Catastrophizing in Combat as Risk and Protection," *Clinical
Psychological Science* 7, no. 3 (January 28, 2019), https://journals.sagepub

.com/doi/10.1177/2167702618813532; Matthew Tull, "Managing Cata-strophic Thinking in PTSD," Verywell Mind, October 24, 2022, https://www.verywellmind.com/managing-catastrophic-thoughts-2797222#citation-2.

4.   Elizabeth Scott, "How Rumination Differs from Emotional Processing," Verywell Mind, September 22, 2022, https://www.verywellmind.com/repetitive-thoughts-emotional-processing-or-rumination-3144936.

PRINCIPLE #2

1.   Richard G. Tedeschi, "Growth After Trauma," *Harvard Business Review*, August 31, 2021, https://hbr.org/2020/07/growth-after-trauma.

2.   Bessel van der Kolk, "Healing from Trauma: Owning Your Self," in *The Body Keeps the Score: Mind, Brain and Body in the Transformation of Trauma* (New York: Penguin, 2015), 208.

PRINCIPLE #3

1.   Tori DeAngelis, "Veterans Are at Higher Risk for Suicide. Psychologists Are Helping Them Tackle Their Unique Struggles," *Monitor on Psychology* 53, no. 8 (November 1, 2022), https://www.apa.org/monitor/2022/11/preventing-veteran-suicide.

2.   Jennifer Kunst, "A Headshrinker's Guide to the Galaxy," *Psychology Today*, September 14, 2011, https://www.psychologytoday.com/us/blog/headshrinkers-guide-the-galaxy.

3.   Toni Benhard, "It's Time to Stop Taking Things Personally," *Psychology Today*, August 28, 2018, https://www.psychologytoday.com/us/blog/turning-straw-gold/201808/its-time-stop-taking-things-personally.

4.   Edith Eva Eger, *The Choice: Embrace the Possible* (New York: Scribner, 2008).

5.   Viktor Frankl, *Man's Search for Meaning* (Boston: Beacon Press, 2016).

6. Rahav Gabay et al., "The Tendency for Interpersonal Victimhood: The Personality Construct and Its Consequences," *Personality and Individual Differences* 165, no. 15 (October 15, 2020), https://doi.org/10.1016/j.paid.2020.110134.

7. Scott Barry Kaufman, "Unraveling the Mindset of Victimhood," *Scientific American*, June 29, 2020, https://www.scientificamerican.com/article/unraveling-the-mindset-of-victimhood/.

8. Mark Barden, "Father of Sandy Hook Victim Says Joe Biden Has Helped Him Process Grief: 'Common Ground,'" *People*, March 11, 2021, https://people.com/crime/mark-barden-sandy-hook-father-president-biden-helped-process-grief/.

9. Kristin Neff, "Definition and Three Elements of Self-Compassion: Kristin Neff," *Self-compassion*, July 9, 2020, https://self-compassion.org/the-three-elements-of-self-compassion-2/.

10. Neff, "Definition and Three Elements."

11. Neff, "Definition and Three Elements."

12. Laura Hillenbrand, *Unbroken: A World War II Story of Survival, Resilience, and Redemption* (New York: Random House, 2010).

13. Amanda Ann Gregory, "Why Forgiveness Isn't Required in Trauma Recovery," *Psychology Today*, February 20, 2022, https://www.psychologytoday.com/us/blog/simplifying-complex-trauma/202202/why-forgiveness-isn-t-required-in-trauma-recovery.

14. Mitch Album, *Tuesdays with Morrie: An Old Man, a Young Man and Life's Greatest Lesson* (New York: Crown, 2002), 166.

PRINCIPLE #4

1. Keti Simmen-Janevska, Veronika Brandstätter, and Andreas Maercker, "The Overlooked Relationship Between Motivational Abilities and Posttraumatic Stress: A Review," *European Journal of Psychotraumatology*

3 (October   31,   2012),   https://www.ncbi.nlm.nih.gov/pmc/articles /PMC3486959/.

2.   Jaime   Booth   Cundy,   "The   Goal   of   Hope,"   *Psychology Today*, May   21,   2011,   https://www.psychologytoday.com/us/blog/the-beauty -in-the-beast/201105/the-goal-hope.

3.   William H. McRaven, *Make Your Bed: Little Things That Can Change Your Life…And Maybe the World* (New York: Grand Central Publishing, 2017).

4.   Geoffrey James, "What Goal-Setting Does to Your Brain and Why It's Spectacularly Effective," Inc., October 23, 2019, https://www.inc.com /geoffrey-james/what-goal-setting-does-to-your-brain-why-its-spectacularly -effective.html; E. A. Locke et al., "Goal Setting and Task Performance: 1969–1980," *Psychological Bulletin* 90, no. 1 (1981): 125–152, https://doi .org/10.1037/0033-2909.90.1.125.

5.   Katy Milkman, *How to Change: The Science of Getting from Where You Are to Where You Want to Be* (New York: Portfolio, 2021).

6.   Katy Milkman, "A Flexible Routine Can Help You Change for Good," Strategy+business, May 6, 2021, https://www.strategy-business .com/article/A-flexible-routine-can-help-you-change-for-good.

7.   Kevin Soong, "6 Simple Steps to Build an Exercise Habit," *Washington Post*, January 2, 2023, https://www.washingtonpost.com /wellness/2023/01/02/exercise-habit-fitness-goals/.

8.   Soong, "6 Simple Steps"; A. D. Mosewich et al., "Self-Compassion: A Potential Resource for Young Women Athletes," *Journal of Sport & Exercise Psychology* 33, no. 1 (2011): 103–123, https://doi.org/10.1123 /jsep.33.1.103.

9.   Tim Blankert and Melvyn R. W. Hamstra, "Imagining Success: Multiple Achievement Goals and the Effectiveness of Imagery," *Basic and Applied Social Psychology* 39, no. 1 (January 2, 2017): 60–67, https:// pubmed.ncbi.nlm.nih.gov/28366970/.

10. Charles Duhigg, *The Power of Habit: Why We Do What We Do in Life and Business* (New York: Random House, 2012).

PRINCIPLE #5

1. Brené Brown, *Atlas of the Heart: Meaningful Connection and the Language of Human Experience* (New York: Random House, 2021).

2. Ioana Pencea et al. "Emotion Dysregulation Is Associated with Increased Prospective Risk for Chronic PTSD Development," *Journal of Psychiatric Research* 121 (February 2020): 222–228, https://www.ncbi.nlm.nih.gov/pmc/articles/PMC6957226/.

3. Annie Tanasugarn, "What Is Emotional Dysregulation, Anyway?" *Psychology Today*, August 26, 2022, https://www.psychologytoday.com/us/blog/understanding-ptsd/202208/what-is-emotional-dysregulation-anyway.

4. Bessel van der Kolk, "Healing from Trauma: Owning Your Self," in *The Body Keeps the Score: Mind, Brain and Body in the Transformation of Trauma* (New York: Penguin, 2015), 208.

5. Van der Kolk, "Healing from Trauma," 209.

6. Marlynn Wei, "New Study Shows Brief Meditation Can Reduce Anger," *Psychology Today*, February 4, 2016, https://www.psychologytoday.com/us/blog/urban-survival/201602/new-study-shows-brief-meditation-can-reduce-anger.

7. "Sympathetic Nervous System (SNS): What It Is & Function," Cleveland Clinic, https://my.clevelandclinic.org/health/body/23262-sympathetic-nervous-system-sns-fight-or-flight.

8. Najma Khorrami, "Gratitude and Its Impact on the Brain and Body," *Psychology Today*, September 4, 2020, https://www.psychologytoday.com/us/blog/comfort-gratitude/202009/gratitude-and-its-impact-the-brain-and-body.

PRINCIPLE #6

1. Rick Hanson, "Taking in the Good vs. the Negativity Bias," accessed March 26, 2023, https://www.sfsu.edu/~holistic/documents/Spring_2014/GoodvsNeg_Bias.pdf.

2 Odelya Gertel Kraybill, "The Neuroscience of Gratitude and Trauma," *Psychology Today*, January 31, 2020, https://www.psychologytoday.com/us/blog/expressive-trauma-integration/202001/the-neuroscience-gratitude-and-trauma.

3. Sunghyon Kyeong et al., "Effects of Gratitude Meditation on Neural Network Functional Connectivity and Brain-Heart Coupling," *Nature News*, July 11, 2017, https://www.nature.com/articles/s41598-017-05520-9.

4. Misty Pratt, "The Science of Gratitude," Mindful, November 10, 2022, https://www.mindful.org/the-science-of-gratitude/.

5. Madhuleena Roy Chowdhury, "The Neuroscience of Gratitude and Effects on the Brain," PositivePsychology.com, April 9, 2023, https://positivepsychology.com/neuroscience-of-gratitude/.

6. NeuroHealth Associates, "Gratitude Literally Rewires Your Brain to Be Happier," July 4, 2022, https://nhahealth.com/neuroscience-reveals-gratitude-literally-rewires-your-brain-to-be-happier/.

7. Andrew Huberman, "The Science of Gratitude & How to Build a Gratitude Practice," Huberman Lab, July 17, 2022, https://hubermanlab.com/the-science-of-gratitude-and-how-to-build-a-gratitude-practice/.

8. Huberman, "The Science of Gratitude."

9. Anderson Cooper, "Stephen Colbert: Grateful for Grief," *All There Is with Anderson Cooper*, September 21, 2022, https://www.cnn.com/audio/podcasts/all-there-is-with-anderson-cooper/episodes/ae2f9ebb-1bc6-4d47-b0f0-af17008dcd0c.

10. Tracy Brower, "Gratitude Is a Key to Happiness: 4 Reasons Why," *Forbes*, November 9, 2022, https://www.forbes.com/sites/tracybrower/2021/04/25/gratitude-is-a-key-to-happiness-4-reasons-why/?sh=6f6d8aeb347c.

11. Eric Pedersen and Debra Lieberman, "How Gratitude Helps Your Friendships Grow," Greater Good, December 6, 2017, https://greatergood.berkeley.edu/article/item/how_gratitude_helps_your_friendships_grow.

PRINCIPLE #7

1. Liz Mineo, "Good Genes Are Nice, but Joy Is Better," *Harvard Gazette*, April 1, 2017, https://news.harvard.edu/gazette/story/2017/04/over-nearly-80-years-harvard-study-has-been-showing-how-to-live-a-healthy-and-happy-life/.

2. Leland Kim, "Loneliness Linked to Serious Health Problems and Death Among Elderly," UC San Francisco, June 18, 2018, https://www.ucsf.edu/news/2012/06/98644/loneliness-linked-serious-health-problems-and-death-among-elderly.

3. Michele M. Kroll, "Prolonged Social Isolation and Loneliness Are Equivalent to Smoking 15 Cigarettes a Day" (blog), University of New Hampshire Extension, May 2, 2022, https://extension.unh.edu/blog/2022/05/prolonged-social-isolation-loneliness-are-equivalent-smoking-15-cigarettes-day.

4. Jill Suttie, "Four Ways Social Support Makes You More Resilient," Greater Good, November 13, 2017, https://greatergood.berkeley.edu/article/item/four_ways_social_support_makes_you_more_resilient.

5. Katie Schultz et al., "Key Roles of Community Connectedness in Healing from Trauma," *Psychology of Violence* 6, no. 1 (January 11, 2017): 42–48, https://pennstate.pure.elsevier.com/en/publications/key-roles-of-community-connectedness-in-healing-from-trauma.

6. "PTSD: National Center for PTSD, "Relationships," US Department of Veterans Affairs, January 1, 2007, https://www.ptsd.va.gov/family/effect_relationships.asp.

7. Tony W. Buchanan et al., "The Empathic, Physiological Resonance of Stress," *Social Neuroscience* 7, no. 2 (July 21, 2011): 191–201, http://www-personal.umich.edu/~prestos/Downloads/BuchananetalSNonline.pdf.

8.   Melody Wilding, "Re-Entry Stress Is Contagious. Here's How to Protect Yourself," *Harvard Business Review*, October 12, 2021, https://hbr.org/2021/10/re-entry-stress-is-contagious-heres-how-to-protect-yourself.

PRINCIPLE #8

1.   Lillian Cunningham, interview with Brené Brown, *The Washington Post on Leadership* (podcast), August 21, 2015, https://www.washingtonpost.com/news/on-leadership/wp/2015/08/21/podcast-brene-brown-on-getting-past-setbacks/.

2.   Angela Duckworth et al., "Grit: Perseverance and Passion for Long-Term Goals," *Journal of Personality and Social Psychology* 96, no. 2 (January 10, 2007): 1087–1101, https://pubmed.ncbi.nlm.nih.gov/17547490/.

PRINCIPLE #9

1.   Marissa Shapiro, "Neuroscientists at Vanderbilt Identify the Brain Cells That Help Humans Adapt to Change," Vanderbilt University, July 15, 2020, https://news.vanderbilt.edu/2020/07/15/neuroscientists-at-vanderbilt-identify-the-brain-cells-that-help-humans-adapt-to-change/.

2.   Kendra Cherry, "Why Our Brains Are Hardwired to Focus on the Negative," Verywell Mind, November 14, 2022, https://www.verywellmind.com/negative-bias-4589618.

3.   Crystal Raypole, "How Many Thoughts Do You Have per Day? and Other Faqs," Healthline Media, February 28, 2022, https://www.healthline.com/health/how-many-thoughts-per-day#thoughts-per-day.

4.   Nancy Colier, "Negative Thinking: A Dangerous Addiction," *Psychology Today*, April 15, 2019, https://www.psychologytoday.com/us/blog/inviting-monkey-tea/201904/negative-thinking-dangerous-addiction.

5.   Kate Hassett, "The Science of Negative Thoughts and How to Stop Them," MiNDFOOD, June 23, 2017, https://www.mindfood.com/article/the-science-of-negative-thoughts-and-how-to-stop-them/.

6. MGH News and Public Affairs, "Mindfulness Meditation Study Shows Changes in Neural Responses to Pain and Fear," *Harvard Gazette*, October 15, 2019, https://news.harvard.edu/gazette/story/2019/10/mindfulness-meditation-study-shows-changes-in-neural-responses-to-pain-and-fear/.

7. "Keep Your Brain Young with Music," Johns Hopkins Medicine, April 13, 2022, https://www.hopkinsmedicine.org/health/wellness-and-prevention/keep-your-brain-young-with-music.

8. Jonah Lehrer, "The Neuroscience of Music," *Wired*, January 19, 2011, https://www.wired.com/2011/01/the-neuroscience-of-music/.

9. Shahram Heshmat, "6 Ways Music Can Reduce Your Stress," *Psychology Today*, October 10, 2022, https://www.psychologytoday.com/us/blog/science-choice/202210/6-ways-music-can-reduce-your-stress.

10. Gabriel Lopez-Garrido, "Self-Efficacy Theory in Psychology: Definition & Examples," Simply Psychology, February 13, 2023, https://www.simplypsychology.org/self-efficacy.html.

11. Cathy Cassata, "Believing You Can Improve Your Mental Well-Being Works," Verywell Mind, July 31, 2022, https://www.verywellmind.com/believing-you-can-improve-your-mental-well-being-helps-5536948.

PRINCIPLE #10

1. E. M.Anicich et al., "Getting Back to the 'New Normal': Autonomy Restoration During a Global Pandemic," *Journal of Applied Psychology* 105, no. 9 (2020), 931–943, https://doi.org/10.1037/apl0000655.

2. Kristin Neff, "The Physiology of Self-Compassion," *Self*, February 22, 2015, https://self-compassion.org/the-physiology-of-self-compassion.

3. Jaime Rosenberg, "The Effects of Chronic Fear on a Person's Health," AJMC, November 11, 2017, https://www.ajmc.com/view/the-effects-of-chronic-fear-on-a-persons-health.

PRINCIPLE #11

1. Ken Falke and Josh Goldberg, *Struggle Well: Thriving in the Aftermath of Trauma* (Carson City, NV: Lioncrest Publishing, 2018).

2. Lorna Collier, "Growth After Trauma," *Monitor on Psychology* 47, no. 10 (November 2016), https://www.apa.org/monitor/2016/11/growth-trauma.

PRINCIPLE #12

1. Eva M. Krackow, "How Many Decisions Do We Make Each Day?" *Psychology Today*, September 27, 2018, https://www.psychologytoday.com/us/blog/stretching-theory/201809/how-many-decisions-do-we-make-each-day.

2. Geoffrey James, "What Goal-Setting Does to Your Brain and Why It's Spectacularly Effective," Inc., October 23, 2019, https://www.inc.com/geoffrey-james/what-goal-setting-does-to-your-brain-why-its-spectacularly-effective.html.

3. Gail Matthews, "The Impact of Commitment, Accountability, and Written Goals on Goal Achievement," Dominican Scholar, 87th Convention of the Western Psychological Association, 2007, https://scholar.dominican.edu/psychology-faculty-conference-presentations/3/.

4. Shane J. Lopez, Jennifer Teramoto Pedrotti, and C. R. Snyder, *Positive Psychology: The Scientific and Practical Explorations of Human Strengths* (Los Angeles: SAGE, 2010).

5. Nicholas A. Kuiper, "Humor and Resiliency: Towards a Process Model of Coping and Growth," *Europe's Journal of Psychology* 8, no. 3 (August 29, 2012): 475–491, https://ejop.psychopen.eu/index.php/ejop/article/view/464.

6. Margaret M. Hansen, Reo Jones, and Kirsten Tocchini, "Shinrin-Yoku (Forest Bathing) and Nature Therapy: A State-of-the-Art Review," *International Journal of Environmental Research and Public Health* 14,

no. 8 (July 28, 2017): 851, https://www.ncbi.nlm.nih.gov/pmc/articles /PMC5580555/.

7. Mathew P. White et al., "Spending at Least 120 Minutes a Week in Nature Is Associated with Good Health and Wellbeing," *Scientific Reports* no. 7730 (2019), https://doi.org/10.1038/s41598-019-44097-3.

8. Nicole J. Hegberg, Jasmeet P. Hayes, and Scott M. Hayes. "Exercise Intervention in PTSD: A Narrative Review and Rationale for Implementation," *Frontiers in Psychiatry* 10 (March 21, 2019): 33, https://www.ncbi.nlm.nih.gov/pmc/articles/PMC6437073/.

9. Melissa J. McGranahan and Patrick J. O'Connor. "Exercise Training Effects on Sleep Quality and Symptoms of Anxiety and Depression in Post-Traumatic Stress Disorder: A Systematic Review and Meta-Analysis of Randomized Control Trials," *Mental Health and Physical Activity* 20 (March 2021), https://www.sciencedirect.com/science/article/abs/pii /S1755296621000053.

10. Annahita S. Irani, "Positive Altruism: Helping That Benefits Both the Recipient and Giver," Capstone Project Master of Applied Positive Psychology, University of Pennsylvania, August 25, 2018, https://core.ac .uk/download/pdf/219379106.pdf.

11. Karen J. Reivich, Martin E. P. Seligman, and Sharon McBride, "Master Resilience Training in the U.S. Army," *American Psychologist*, January 2011, https://pubmed.ncbi.nlm.nih.gov/21219045/.

12. Lindsey R. Monger, "Hunting the Good Stuff During Resiliency Training," US Army, January 5, 2015, https://www.army.mil/article/140671 /hunting_the_good_stuff_during_resiliency_training; Robert A. Emmons, *Thanks!: How the New Science of Gratitude Can Make You Happier* (Boston: Houghton Mifflin Harcourt, 2007).

ABOUT THE AUTHOR

Staff Sergeant Travis Mills (US Army, Retired) is a recalibrated warrior, motivational speaker to corporations worldwide, actor, author, and advocate for veterans and amputees. He and his wife, Kelsey, founded the Travis Mills Foundation, a nonprofit organization formed to benefit and assist veterans. Mills continues to speak all over the country. He lives in Maine with his wife and two children, Chloe and Dax.